Real Movement

PERSPECTIVE ON INTEGRATED MOTION & MOTOR CONTROL

As a practitioner I am all about the 'why'. Courses and books aimed at the 'how' are fine, but for me, understanding why you're doing something in the first place, or why a patient is experiencing something in the first place is the most important part of any treatment. To that end, one could say that with its central theme of 'why', this book answers the most important 'how' question posed by any practitioner: How do I best help my patients? For those folks still craving some tangible 'how-to's' Adam does provide a nice section of clinical pearls at the end of the book, however, he never strays from his unstated philosophy of 'treat the human, not just the tissue.' It doesn't focus solely on one approach, one technique, or one concept. You get a little bit of Anatomy Trains, a little bit of Gray Institute, a little bit of NKT, a dash of FRC, and a whole lot of Adam Wolf.--**C. Shante Cofield, PT, DPT, OCS,**

www.TheMovementMaestro.com

"Whenever I'm around Adam, I find myself craving more information and insights into how he views the human body. Real Movement gave me a glimpse into the unique and vast knowledge that Adam possesses about how we move and has allowed me to learn from him over and over again, even when I'm not physically in his presence. The human machine is wonderfully complex, which allows us to do everything that we love to do, but can also make treating it exhausting. By combining the principles of motor control, stability, fascia, and gait into easily understood and applied concepts and case studies, Adam has made this is a must read text for anyone who works with the human body." **Mitch Hauschildt, MA, ATC, CSCS, Missouri State University, Prevention, Rehab and Physical Performance Coordinator**

"Whether you are a skilled clinician, new graduate or just someone who is passionate about the human body, Adam Wolf is a person you should absolutely have on your list of people to learn from. With all of the debate on what movement is and should be, Adam provides an evidence-informed approach with a fresh and eye opening take on what's Real. As a clinician and self-proclaimed movement geek, this book has allowed me to expand on my knowledge and feel comfortable implementing new strategies that are outside of the box, functional and highly effective." **Rick Daigle, PT, DPT, FMT-C, STMT-1, Owner, Medical Minds In Motion,**

www.MedicalMindsInMotion.com

Real Movement

PERSPECTIVE ON INTEGRATED MOTION & MOTOR CONTROL

Adam Wolf, PT, LMT, FAFS

Golden Mango Press

Golden Mango Press is an imprint of Green Tomato Publishing. LLC.

Real Movement: Perspective on Integrated Motion & Motor Control/ Adam Wolf. —1st ed.
ISBN-13: 978-0692811955
ISBN-10: 0692811958

To my beautiful children, Alexia and Elijah. I love you.

"Learning is not a product of schooling, but the lifelong attempt to acquire it."

—Albert Einstein

Contents

Foreword by Dr. Gary Gray, PT, FAFS 1

Preface 3

Introduction... 9

Chapter 1:   The Interconnectedness of the Body.................................. 17

Chapter 2:   Movement & Fascial Connections 23

Chapter 3:   3-Dimensional Movement Defined 29

Chapter 4:   Motor Control Theories and Their Importance in 3D Movement 47

Chapter 5:   Integration of Fascia & Nervous System............................ 55

Chapter 6:   Injury 63

Chapter 7:   Composition of Tissue & Scars.. 77

Clinical Considerations.. 85

Chapter 8:   Clinical Considerations for the Lower Extremity.............................. 87

Chapter 9:   Clinical Considerations for Thoracic Spine & Upper Extremity... 115

Chapter 10:   Exercise Library 133

Chapter 11:   Conclusion 165

Bibliography.. 169

Acknowledgements 173

FOREWORD

One of the greatest gifts we can possess as we grow and develop in any profession is the gift of discerning synthesis. Adam Wolf reveals his giftedness of judgment and understanding along with unification and integration within his book entitled *Real Movement*. Throughout this text we get the privilege of journeying with Adam through his own personal development as a movement professional. The gift of this book is about the wisdom revealed by Adam with his ability to discern and synthesize all that he has been exposed to in this complex field of human movement. Being influenced by numerous books, articles, seminars, videos and individuals (most notably and proudly his father) Adam shares his insightful intellect along with his ability to blend and fuse as evidenced in this book. The result is an easy to ready, easy to understand, common sense approach to facilitating "real movement" - the right movement at the right time for the right purpose for all individuals.

You will enjoy many of his analogies, especially the seven oceans versus the one ocean used to correlate with appreciating the body in isolation versus the body as an integrated system. Adam gives clarity to our need to comprehend and take advantage of motor control theories, with an emphasis on the ultimate driver of all movement, the nervous system. By pulling out KEY CONCEPT in each section, along with practical clinical considerations, there is significant added value to the text. Case studies, always a powerful way to reveal the why behind the what, are included to reinforce the strategies presented.

Adam has learned, and eloquently shares this wisdom with us, that there is no one best solution to human movement disorders. He teaches us the value of discernment of the many approaches that are available to us. As important, we benefit from his ability to synthesize the best approaches to a practical blend of techniques to create the most optimal environments for each individual.

Perhaps the most significant truth revealed in this book is how much Adam is in love with his profession, and as a result how much his profession is in love with him. May we take advantage of this love, and may we continue to grow in our purpose and passion of serving others as we read, enjoy, and practice in *Real Movement*.

Dr. Gary Gray, PT, FAFS

CEO, Gray Institute & creator of "Applied Functional Science"

As a student of integrated motion before PT school, it was a continual source of study during my formal PT education, despite not being part of the program curriculum. Reconciling the information became challenging because teachers would say a muscle does one thing, IE extend the knee in isolation in one plane of motion, while my outside education demonstrated exactly the opposite. The quadriceps can perform knee extension, but from an integrated lens, controls the knee from flexing (abducting and internally rotating) when the foot hits the ground (for lunging, squatting, walking, running), together with the tissue above and below, in all three planes of motion. Attempting to discuss this knowledge with peers and teachers was, at times, frustrating, because I was learning about the body from two seemingly different sources. When I would question this paradoxical situation, the response typically was, and still is, "where's the research?"

As I've continued taking and teaching courses, and I do a fair amount of both, there isn't any one resource to go to, and there shouldn't be. Yet, practically every time I teach, there are inquiries for further information on the topics we covered, specifically movement and motor control principles, and where it can be found. This work represents my effort to tie all I've learned up to this point that's been clinically relevant, in hopes of being a resource that enhances clinical practice because I've been fortunate to have learned with, and directly from many of the people discussed in this text. My intention is to offer a taste of various thought processes and how I incorporate them into my clinical practice, in order for you to go to the source for a full drink. This work represents the culmination of all of my movement journals organized into one workable body, and my advice while reading this book is find truths to anchor to.

I began my career as a physical therapist in an outpatient sports medicine/orthopedic setting in the South Loop of Chicago, and upon starting my business, supplemented my income working as a contract therapist. This provided an opportunity to work in multiple physical therapy environments, including home health, inpatient and outpatient hospital based PT, nursing homes, assisted living facilities and rehab hospitals treating multiple pathologies. I treated high volumes of patients, and worked with some very talented clinicians, revealing more than one way to treat, and there was a lot to learn. While in these settings, I noticed that overall most clinicians tended to treat only in their respective environments. Outpatient PTs tended to stick to outpatient PT and inpatient, hospital PTs tended to stick with inpatient hospital work, and generally, each respective environment tended to have their "exercises/protocols/ways to treat" relative to that particular environment, without carryover between environments. However through studying integrated motion, I recognized universal truths, regardless of environment, despite the disconnect.

My formal education taught to be an entry level clinician, not hurt anybody, and confirmed that how we learn about the body is often disjointed. In retrospect, I'm most grateful that I learned *how* to learn, while also learning what they taught me. The concept of lifelong learning was instilled in me by a professor, Dr. Margaret Plack, who at the time was the Director of the George Washington University Physical Therapy department, where I received my physical therapy degree. This perspective of lifelong learning, combined with an understanding of how I learn has been a focus professionally.

I learn best by being able to first read about a concept, then observe it and be able to ask questions is how I retain the most information. I need to see how and why the concept is used for me to translate it into something workable in my practice. For this reason, the concept of parampara has helped me personally and professionally. Parampara is a Sanskrit word that translates to "an uninterrupted row or series, succession, and continuation of knowledge (in any field) that is passed down through successive generations. Examples include spiritually, artistic, music, dance or education." Once I learned about this concept, shortly after beginning a yoga practice for exercise and stress relief, it fascinated me. Etiology has always been of interest, and when I became aware that yoga was traditionally taught individually from teacher to student, a philosophy I already practiced, I wanted to learn more. In retrospect, I've taken many classes and learned *from* many people, but my true teachers are those that I've learned from both in a group environment and also *with* them one on one. At this point in each area of my learning, I can say that I have a teacher to guide me through questions and sticking points.

Early on, one such teacher, and now friend, Lenny Parracino, recommended keeping a journal of truths to write down concepts that I could anchor to while learning. He also advised me that when learning about a topic, to read a lot of sources from many viewpoints. I divided part of my 'movement journal' into a "physical truths" section, "biological truths" section, and "behavioral truths" section, which aligned perfectly with the concepts of Applied Functional Science (AFS), which I was studying intently at the time. AFS is defined as the integration of the physical, biological and behavioral sciences, and once I began learning this way, found it very easy to read and extract, while also identifying what was being said that didn't align. I still do this, although less formally, as evidenced in my notes in any course I ever attend. What's typically written down are concepts that fit into one of these buckets.

KEY CONCEPT: I found it helpful for my learning to keep a section of my learning journal for 'truth's'. My journal was divided into a physical truths section, biological truths section, and behavioral truths section. With this journal, when reading anything, I would search for and anchor to the truths, relative to that topic. This approach has helped me to integrate various thoughts and 'ways' of doing things typically designated by capital letters after someone's title (i.e. AFS, NKT, ART, FMT, FRC, FMS, etc.) which all are systems that have truths that unite them.

With consistent strategies in place, I felt freed from constraints in each treatment environment. For me, continuing to learn new things and concepts is the key for synthesizing and creating more neural connections. My learnings have drifted from specifically physical therapy and movement topics to more abstract topics in behavior, mindfulness, yoga, and music. Currently I'm learning the guitar, which has proven exciting, difficult, and also meditative. I feel more relaxed after, and appreciate that everything just described creates stimulation in my brain, producing myelination and new pathways. It also reinforces old pathways and perpetuates the feedback loop to be able to synthesize information, which for me is a desired trait.

KEY CONCEPT: We need stimulation for myelination. Learning new things is stimulating, and creates new connections in the brain via neuroplasticity. An old dog can learn new tricks.

For me, the request "where's the research" sometimes feels contradictory. Some things are difficult to prove through research, yet it doesn't mean it isn't true or applicable. After all, how would someone know what to research if it wasn't first correlated without research? Often times, a conversation around movement begins and progresses in one of two directions, depending on willingness to consider concepts one perhaps never before conceptualized. While I try and stay up to date and read current research, truthfully, I don't feel intelligent enough to fully understand a lot of it and recently have begun to feel turned off by the recent dominance of research over clinical experience in some movement circles. I rely on friends and colleagues that are smarter to direct me to good research, in each of the 'communities' I have professional contact with. Like anything I read professionally, as long as there are truths to anchor to, there will be relevance, while also trying to recognize my cognitive biases towards certain topics.

Relative to speaking to people in the movement industry, it boils down to the following: either the person is or isn't willing to accept the basic premise that the body, governed by the nervous system, and is an integrated unit that desires lengthening and accepting load prior to shortening and producing force whenever possible. In the book *Mindset*, Dr. Carol Dweck describes a fixed versus growth mindset. A fixed mindset as one that "assumes that our character, intelligence and creative abilities are static givens which can't change in any meaningful way", while a growth mindset "thrives on challenge and sees failure not as evidence of unintelligence, but as a heartening springboard for growth and for stretching our existing abilities."

Insight into someone's mindset has proven beneficial when interacting with people, and I've observed that most times behavior change is required when someone is in pain. Therefore, perspective on mindset about a person's pain and daily routine is useful. Sometimes that behavior change is someone knowing when in a bad position for extended periods, in order to not do that, potentially lessening the stress to a particular tissue. Other times, the behavior change is in recognizing when their self-talk or thoughts aren't serving them, potentially creating and reinforcing the sympathetic nature already likely being perpetuated. People with a fixed mindset typically have an internal dialogue full of judgement, where there is constant measurement, versus people with an open mindset, which tend to have dialogue about observing, learning, improving, and getting better. Most times, first sessions with me include recognizing which behavior needs to change in order to produce the positive, feed forward mechanism necessary for getting better.

When a behavior is a driver of pain, in order to make change, awareness must first be drawn to the specific behavior and how it could potentially be contributing to a pain cycle. Clinical experience demonstrates that typically people in pain are unaware of the behavior that may be a contributor. Simply put, they don't know they don't know, and breath work can be a useful tool in creating behavior change. The act of inhaling and exhaling, ideally through the nose with long slow exhales, stimulates parasympathetic response necessary to create change in the nervous system, while bringing awareness to whatever is identified. The act of breathing is conscious, versus respirating, which is a subconscious act of oxygen exchange that is a natural process. When a distinction is made between respiration and breathing, the very tool of the breath can be utilized to aid in behavior change.

Clinically, the most beneficial breathing techniques I use in my clinical practice often come straight from the fourth limb of yoga, pranayama. I've learned many techniques from the person I consider to be my yoga teacher in Chicago, Jim Bennitt, educator and co-owner of Tejas Yoga in Chicago. Yoga, while often identified as an exercise, can also be a lifestyle and philosophy on life. Personally and professionally yoga has made positive impact on numerous levels. Simply put, I've found many yoga exercises very beneficial, and when applied scientifically and specifically, can enhance both mobility and motor control. I appreciate how each movement can be linked with either an inhalation or exhalation, and that the practice became so much harder, deeper, and more meaningful when the breath was focused on during an entire movement. Jim instilled for me the understanding that the breath should be long, slow, through the nose whenever possible, and should last slightly longer than the movement. The inability to breathe during a movement is indicative of compensation of the nervous system.

I observe that most times, if something is difficult, physically or emotionally, the breath is held. If we can identify those instances, and can breathe long and slow, often a physiological and energetic softening will be felt. My belief is this flow of breath is a key to becoming more aware. Personally, taking a breath before acting has allowed me to better observe myself, and awareness of self in any environment, i.e. while sitting at your workstation at the computer or standing in line at the grocery store, can allow you to become aware of your positioning and how it might be leading to your pain or dysfunction. This awareness can also be useful in situations where reacting instead of responding is regrettable. During movement, muscles reacting is preferable, but for the conscious self, responding is preferable to reacting. This is another paradox of life, because in movement we react; however, responding consciously provides us a choice.

Reacting is an internal stimulus, and responding is an external, or conscious, spur to act. Behaviorally, I feel it's best to respond instead of react. Admittedly, I struggle with this, and responding instead of reacting is something I continue to focus on personally. I feel grateful that my mindset and way I've chosen to live my life allows me to practice continually. On a regular basis, I practice the art and science of physical therapy and yoga. I get to practice the guitar and especially practice being a better father, friend and partner. Admittedly I'm not as good at any of it as I'd like to be, but I reckon that's why it's called a practice.

KEY CONCEPT: Reacting is a stimulus versus responding, which is an external, or conscious, spur to act.

I encourage you to find a central place to synthesize all relevant concepts, and to divide them into the various buckets, especially when reading this book. It represents my current and present level of understanding, awareness, and ability to synthesize some of the information presented. I recognize that each of the topics discussed could be and is a book in itself, and by no means is the final word on anything discussed. It's my attempt at anchoring to truths. I advise drinking many flavors of the proverbial Kool-Aid, and I encourage you, the reader, to synthesize information, anchor to truths, and create your way based on sound principles.

INTRODUCTION

Healers have learned and written about the body for thousands of years, including "Internal Classics" written by Chinese scholars as early as 475 B.C. and the Yoga Sutras of Patanjali, written over 2000 years ago. The Yin-Yang doctrine and the theory of circulation are thought processes that came out of these works, while the Greek philosopher Hippocrates was the first person to separate medicine from magic in 400 BC. Aristotle wrote that the heart was the focus of blood vessels, while other examples of soft tissue work being integrated into movement therapies include Yoga and Ayurvedic medicine as well as the Vedas, written in 1500 B.C. Of specific interest for me is the self-tissue work abhyanga, Sanskrit for self-oil massage, as the benefits and improvement of both physiological and energetic "flow" were seen thousands of years ago and only now are being re-recognized for their importance and ability to decrease pain and increase vitality.

Traditionally, movement professionals in the West have learned about the body in a systems-driven, isolated perspective. While this method is vital in our understanding of how the body is put together, the reality it's far more complex because the body works as an integrated unit works together and nothing exists in isolation. This isolated mentality of the West is beginning to be replaced with what is considered to be more an Eastern mindset, one of integration where it's recognized that the site of the injury isn't the cause of the injury, accurately reflected by Ida Rolf when she said, "Where you think it is, it ain't."

I came to love movement early, playing multiple sports as a youth. I began my career as a physical therapy aide at the National Rehabilitation Hospital in Washington, DC, also working as a personal trainer while completing the 5 classes required to begin PT school. This was an important experience because I worked with very high level functioning individuals and also very low level function directly alongside experienced clinicians treating a variety of pathologies within the movement spectrum. I had an early advantage because my father, Chuck Wolf, is an educator in the fitness industry and exposed me to his work early on. I began studying and learning his work, practicing with my personal training clients. This led me to Dr. Gary Gray, PT and the 3 dimensional movement of Applied Functional Science (AFS) which is the lens in which I view every other modality. Except for a brief break during PT school to learn what the test was teaching, AFS has been a continuous source of study and undoubtedly a differentiator as a clinician.

Yet early in my career I was left wondering if the work I was doing was working or not. Certainly a piece was clinical experience, but why would two people with the exact same symptoms and pathology have two drastically different outcomes? I couldn't satisfactorily answer, which led me to search for more tools that could help me find answers. It took approximately 5 years, and I finally felt I found an answer through Dr. Nicholas Studholme, a chiropractor and movement geek out of Denver, Colorado, who also completed a Fellowship of Applied Functional Science through the Gray Institute. The Gray Institute is led by Dr. Gray, which is where I obtained my Fellowship in Applied Functional Science (FAFS), and solidified my approach to movement. Dr. Studholme uses a variety of muscle-testing techniques combined with integrated movement in his practice. Up until that point, I had dismissed muscle testing because it seemed virtually at the other end of the spectrum versus AFS because AFS teaches that the body does not know what a muscle is (it's a manmade construct) and that it knows how to control movement. Integrated motions where the body controls the forces presented to it, instead of isolated muscles working to create a movement. In retrospect, I demonstrated confirmation bias, thinking there was no truth behind muscle testing because why would I test a muscle if they don't really exist? However after conversations with colleagues and mentors, combined with having a couple individuals (including Dr. Studholme) demonstrate how they integrate muscle-testing with integrated movement, I realized these two seemingly very different thought processes could actually be blended together in order to choose what 3 dimensional movement will be most effective.

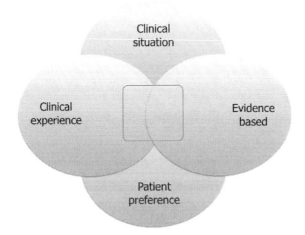

EBP is the integration of clinical expertise, patient values, and the best research evidence into the decision making process for patient care. Clinical expertise refers to the clinician's cumulated experience, education and clinical skills. The patient brings to the encounter his or her own personal preferences and unique concerns, expectations, and values. The best research evidence is usually found in clinically relevant research that has been conducted using sound methodology. (Sackett D, 2002)

This led to investigating further the tool of muscle testing, which I found popular in the Chiropractic and Massage Therapy worlds, but less so in the Physical Therapy or rehab fields because, like AFS, is a difficult subject to prove or disprove. Consequently, western medicine and particularly the physical therapy world has been slower to adopt these methodologies, as these disciplines are so biased towards research in their clinical approach. Yet they both make sense intuitively when you experience them and at the same time, discovered Dr.Sackett, who is the father of evidenced based medicine, and his guide to clinical decision making. It states that only 10% of decision making is evidenced based, and the majority is clinical experience, situation and preference.

Research is clear that with injury there is an inhibited and delayed muscle timing, and there is also a protective mechanism that increases flexor tone and inhibits extensor tone. Why know it exists and do nothing about it? Prior to muscle testing I'm not sure I was doing much to understand if my clients demonstrated these relationships. Since then I've concluded there are numerous ways to assess muscles inhibitions, with the point being to open a neurological window in order to change the aberrant afferent input while using authentic movement as a guide.

Mark Twain said, "There is no such thing as a new idea. It is impossible. We simply take a lot of old ideas and put them into a sort of mental kaleidoscope. We give them a turn and they make new and curious combinations. We keep on turning and making new combinations indefinitely; but they are the same old pieces of colored glass that have been in use through all the ages." It is with this spirit that I offer the reader this work, which is my interpretation of others work, as nothing is new. This text is simply a reflection of the kaleidoscope of my brain at this point in my life and will undoubtedly be tweaked and progressed as I am tweaked and progress.

I recognize that there are weekend courses that total hundreds of hours on each of the topics discussed, including movement, bodywork, and muscle-testing. This book is simply to introduce concepts and serve as a stepping stone to learn more about each respective discipline.

This work presents my present understanding about how the nervous system works, and how using three dimensional movement can be authentically blended with many other techniques to create an authentic and effective movement sessions. This book isn't meant to be the definitive voice on anything, rather to serve as a guide in ways to enhance the quality of movement and, therefore, the quality of life of those we serve. I have been, and am apprehensive to put my thoughts down in this manner. However, my experiences teaching other movement based practitioners, including PTs, OTs, DCs, PTAs, COTAs, MDs, DOs, Osteopaths and personal trainers has made me realize that what I assume is common knowledge isn't.

There is one ocean, not seven. Seven oceans is a manmade construct, just as the concept of isolated muscles is manmade. It's possible to dissect out individual muscles and classify them into isolated groups that work separately to produce forces through a concentric shortening. Yet in reality our nervous system regulates and controls forces while tissues lengthen to control gravity, ground reaction, mass, momentum, and other forces presented. For example, an integrated approach strives to incorporate multiple joints and planes into a movement in order to functionally stretch the abdominals, because it's important that hip flexors be lengthened with the abdominals. Hip flexor flexibility adds to the motion of the abdominals and torso extension in the sagittal plane. When dynamic extension actions occur, which happens during gait, the abdominals and hip flexors must be able to accommodate adequate excursion to perform optimally.

Like the childhood rhyme says, the hip bone's connected to the head bone, via a bunch of other bones and through myofascia. This integrated approach considers the source of symptoms and also understands that the area of pain is NOT necessarily the cause, although it can be. Potential sources of the symptom could emanate from local structures under the area of pain, or remote structures capable of referring pain to the area such as a joint, spinal level, or other muscles connected through fascia to the same kinetic chain. Other contributing factors that could exacerbate pain, such as structural, biomechanical, environmental or behavioral contributors, also must be considered, all of which will be discussed in later sections.

Book Overview

Originally, this book began as an exercise of putting together a 'self-release' and exercise manual for my clients, with the thought of preventing tissue insult. However, as I continued developing as a clinician, so did the concept for the original book. My clinical experience has led me to believe that more often we effect the software, or nervous system, rather than the hardware, or actual structure of the body while working with clients, although there are many instances where the structure is the driver of dysfunction. In other words, structural changes occur in tissue less often than neurological changes, and at the very least most times it's the neurological changes that influence structural change. I believe that most times, what we're doing is changing the perception and connection with a region of the body rather than changing actual tissue. Reprogramming the perception of the aberrant afferents, yet there are many times when we need to change the tissue to make the nervous system function more efficient.

In creating this text, I had difficulty finding anything that combines the thought of true integrated movement in the context of a neurological, Motor Control perspective. In fact, there is very little in literature on true integrated movement at all, while the majority of literature on Motor Control approaches movement from an isolated, muscle instead of an integrated perspective.

Having said that, this book isn't designed to be the comprehensive, final word on any of the subjects discussed, and continues to be a work in progress. Rather, my objective has become to meld various thought processes into a workable format, one that has been successful for me as a clinician and my many thousands of clients. My hope is that you will find this text useful in your own work or personal practice. Undoubtedly it's a work in progress, and so the book you read before you today will be much different in a few years as it, and I, progress.

Chapter 1 will discuss the interconnectedness of the body and discuss the basic thought process of how to address the "why". While putting this material together, I realized there isn't much continuity of words across professions.

Chapter 2 introduces specific fascial connections and motions they control, while *Chapter 3* defines the principles of three dimensional, integrated joint motion from a thought process that bones move, joints feel, and muscles react to movement. This concept, along with an understanding of where and how movement is created, will be elaborated on.

Chapter 4 discusses Motor Control theories, and the motor cortex and cerebellum's role in regulating movement. The concepts of facilitations and inhibition will be introduced, as well as reciprocal inhibitions relative to three dimensional movement.

Chapter 5 discusses how limitations in movement will often result in restrictions in movement away from the site of injury. There will also be a discussion of strategies to increase tissue mobility and extensibility utilizing principles of motor control. The discussion of fascia and how it often is the intersection of the motor and nervous systems comprises *Chapter 6*.

Chapter 7 offers perspective on injuries in general, while discussing the cumulative injury/negative feedback/inflammatory cycles and Chapters 8-10 will be case study and further clinical considerations.

Who Can Use This Manual?

Movement Professionals including:

- Physical Therapists
- Chiropractors
- Athletic Trainers
- Massage Therapists
- Yoga, Pilates instructors
- Personal trainers and advanced movement enthusiasts

Why Use This Manual?

The way we've traditionally learned how the body is connected is systems-driven and isolated, and the typical way in which anatomy, physiology, biology, and the rest is from this perspective, despite it being only a partial perspective. As movement professionals, we strive to describe a more true nature in which the body works together, combined with the thought process of specific therapeutic applications of movement to increase function naturally and authentically.

This manual is to be used as a basic guide to a few of the modalities that have worked well together clinically to help people move and feel better, including integrated movement and muscle testing as an insight into the nervous system. The text will discuss fascial connections that exist in the body, particularly within the context of integrated movement, and hopefully will guide learning and where to find more on any of the subjects discussed within. By no means is this designed to be the final word on anything, and at all times will provide my resources for you to learn more directly from the source.

This manual is for the movement enthusiast, professional or recreational, who wants a better understanding of how to take care of their body within this context.

This is for other professionals in other disciplines. My hope is that it can be used to bridge the gap that exists between professions, including Chiropractic, Massage Therapy, Personal Trainers and other movement professionals, and that clients/patients will want to share this work with their providers (and vice versa), to help themselves and spread the NeuroMovement "word" into the world.

How to Use This Manual

This book has been organized into sections that first discuss consistencies of the body and what I feel is the way muscles/tissue tend to work in most upright function, relative to a motor control perspective. In addition to discussing HOW to identify tri-plane motion, the text will discuss strategies to enhance motion and/or stability. The final sections of the book are broken into body sections and discuss some common pathologies associated with each part. There are also movements/assessment techniques and some basic exercises that may be of benefit for that particular diagnosis.

This is NOT a protocol-driven manual where all the answers lie. It is organized basically in the order in which I learned more in-depth about each subject. There is no one way to do anything, and the right way is the one that gets someone feeling better. If we can follow authentic truths of function, combined with clinical acumen, the treatment becomes apparent. I've heard my friend and mentor Dr. Gary Gray PT, Ph.D. say "try and prove yourself wrong," which is an interesting way of making sure you're right. We all have our confirmation bias, and that, combined with a desire to help those we work with, can lead to a situation where our treatments aren't as effective as can be.

CHAPTER 1

The Interconnectedness of the Body

Fascial Connections of the Body

In 1976 Dr. Irwin Korr stated:

"The spinal cord is the keyboard on which the brain plays when it calls for activity. But each 'key' in the console sounds not an individual 'tone' such as the contraction of a particular group of muscle fibers, but a whole 'symphony' of motion. In other words, build into the cord is a large repertoire of patterns of activity, each involving the complex, harmonious, delicately balanced orchestration of the contractions and relaxation of many muscles. The brain thinks in terms of whole motions, not individual muscles. It calls selectively, for the preprogrammed patterns in the cord and brainstem, modifying them in countless ways and combining them in an infinite variety in still more complex patterns. Each activity is subject to further modulation, refinement, and adjustment by the feedback continually streaming in from the participating muscles, tendons and joints" (Chaitow, 2002, p. 33).

The traditional lens in which to view muscles is one of isolation, where the shortening motion is described as the muscle action, and each muscle has a beginning and an end. For example, isolation describes the quadriceps muscle, located in the thigh, as a knee straightener, with the origin (beginning) being the top of the femur and the insertion (end) being the patellar tendon into the tibia. When these two points are brought together, the knee will straighten. Yet this is exactly the opposite of what the quadriceps do when working with other muscles and tissue to control the body as it reacts to the forces continuously presented to it, including gravity, ground forces, mass and momentum. This integrated mindset of tissue controlling forces in order to remain upright and effectively move throughout the day allows a different lens in which to look at muscle action. Through this lens, it's seen that the muscles on the front of the thigh, that we call the quadriceps, in conjunction with other muscles lengthens to control the knee from bending, rather than straightening the knee. When necessary, muscles CAN produce forces in order to create a motion; however, acting upon anything requires a great deal of energy compared to REACTING to the environment in an integrated way that allows proper and efficient control.

The concept of interrelated and interconnected tissues that works together controlling the body allows a better understanding of the true nature of the body. Pioneers in the world of movement, fascia and the intersection of the nervous system, include Robert Schleip, Ida Rolf (developer of Structural Integration), Thomas Myers, and the Stecco family (developers of Fascial Manipulation). Other contributors to how the neurological system integrates with the fascial system include Robert Carrick, Vladimir Janda, and George Goodheart, while in the movement world, pioneers such as Moshe Feldenkrais, Gary Gray, and renowned yogi Krishnamacharya, his son DKT Desikichar and nephew BKS Iyengar are just a few who have contributed to my understanding of the interconnectedness of the body. Although each discipline is unique and different from the other, commonalities can be found between disciplines that demonstrate how the body is connected from top to bottom, inside to out, and in mind, body, and spirit.

There are many examples of fascial connections, including what my father refers to as the "Anterior X-Factor", consisting of tissue on the front of the hip, up through the trunk and into the opposite shoulder and arm musculature. While stretching the upper extremity (i.e., the shoulder joint), it's important to understand what plane of motion the person is trying to increase in the shoulder. From an integrated lens, the hips play an integral role in shoulder function and need to be incorporated movements designed to increase mobility and stability. For example, in the sagittal plane, sufficient hip extension on the same side is necessary for shoulder flexion. In this fascial connection, referred to as the Anterior Flexibility Highway, these respective motions should occur together in order to minimize the risk of shoulder or low back pain. Chuck states,

> "When thinking about the anatomy of each highway, considering the Myofascial attachments of one muscle and the adjacent muscles as interchanges on an interstate highway is helpful. When one muscle or 'street' ends, it conjoins or 'interchanges' with the next muscle or 'street' in order to control the forces (gravity, ground force, mass, momentum) presented." (Flexibility Highways)

For example, while reading this at home, stand up as tall as possible, with feet at shoulder distance apart. Now, take your right hand and reach overhead behind as far as possible without allowing your pelvis to translate anterior. Take note of how far you could reach behind before pain, discomfort, pinch in the low back, or end-range. Now, keep your hand where it is (flexed overhead) and step your left foot forward, and notice how much range of motion (ROM) exists in the right shoulder with the same side hip in extension, as opposed to a neutral position. There is more, or there should be.

This is applicable for the person who has anterior shoulder impingement, perhaps when they reach up to put dishes into the cabinet from the dishwasher. Perhaps this is the person who has increased kyphosis, or maybe a large lumbar lordosis (or both). If they are unable to achieve hip extension while reaching overhead, the resultant motion will be less spinal exten-sion and less posterior tilt of the scapula, potentially causing impingement of the anterior shoulder tissue with flexion activities. However, if the hip is able to go through extension, the spine will react to the motion below and go through extension, which allows the scapula to tilt backwards and clear room for the humerus to reach overhead without impingement.

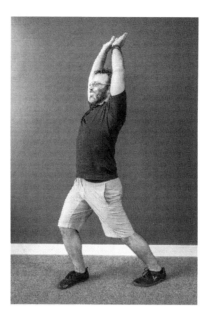

Hip extension creates lumbar and thoracic exten-sion, allowing posterior scapular tilt and decreases the chance of the shoulder muscles impinging be-tween the humeral head and the acromion process due to lack of proper shoulder complex function.

KEY CONCEPT: when stretching the shoulder it is important to incorporate the hips into a stretch, because they work together.

Caroline Stone, Osteopath and author of Science in the Art of Osteopathy, states that hu-man form is "in reality a compromise between the ideal and the actual" (p. 98). The fact that the structure has to be multifunctional means that, for each separate individual function arising from the same structure, the form of the structure may not be ideal. In this way, structure places some constraints/limits on function. This indicates a reciprocal relationship between structure and function, which is an important theme within movement therapies.

Sue Falsone, Doctor of Physical Therapy and Certified Athletic Trainer eloquently stated:

"Manual therapy is all about improving structure. We know we are not going to change or remold bone, but we are attempting to change whatever soft tissue structures we can. We attempt to lengthen, stabilize, impact physiological healing and change, mold and adapt soft tissue. Our structure is going to dictate the function of the area...Why is the glenohumeral 'ball and socket' shaped differently than the femoroacetabular 'ball and socket'? The shoulders are built for more mobility for the needs of the upper extremity while the hip joints need more structural stability to carry our body. Structure dictates function...Function will eventually dictate structure...Structure and function go hand in hand and cannot be separated" (Falsone, May 13, 2014).

It's undeniable that structure and function are interconnected, and it can be seen throughout many professions. For example, offensive linemen in football are going to be very large individuals, as their structure directly dictates their ability to function as a lineman. Another example are manual therapists, who tend to have well-developed hand muscles, or dentists that have increased thoracic kyphosis, while old blues guitarists have crooked fingers as a result of the countless hours of their hands being in that specific position, or dentists with hyper-kyphotic thoracic curves as a result of hours of working in mouths.

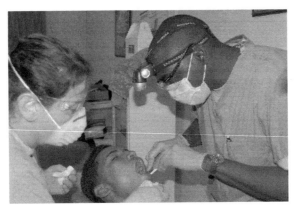

Structure and function are interrelated, as evidenced in the posture, based on positioning, of a dentist. The majority of dentists have increased thoracic kyphosis based on the nature of their work.

In swing sport and rotational athletes, including baseball, tennis, and golf, participants tend to have overly developed spinal erectors on one side versus the other as the result of so much forceful rotation in one direction. In each example, one's function dictates their structure, and vice versa.

Additional Reading Suggestions

Chaitow, L. *Muscle energy techniques*. Edinburgh: Churchill Livingstone/Elsevier.

Falsone, S. *East vs. West* | Structure & Function. www.suefalsone.com

Rolf, Ida P. *Rolfing: Reestablishing the Natural Alignment and Structural Integration of the Human Body for Vitality and Well-being*. Rochester, VT: Healing Arts, 1989. Print.

Myers, Thomas W. *Anatomy Trains: Myofascial Meridians for Manual and Movement Therapists*. Edinburgh: Churchill Livingstone, 2001. Print.

Desikachar, T. K. *The heart of yoga: Developing a personal practice*. Rochester, VT: Inner Traditions International.

Gray, G. *Functional Video Digest Series*. Vol 1.1 the Knee, Vol 2.11 Functional Flexibility

CHAPTER 2

Movement & Fascial Connections

There are numerous ways to name the connections of muscles and fascia, and perhaps the most well-known is described in the book Anatomy Trains by Thomas Myers. However, the concept of interrelated fascial connections are evident through many professions, including most Fascial Manipulation, developed by the Stecco's in Italy and Functional Range Release developed by Dr. Andreo Spina, DC, in Canada. Up until recently, anatomical education focused on a structural and mechanical understanding of individualized human structures, such as muscles, nerves, ligaments, and organs. These 'myofascial lines' have become more prominent in the movement industry as scientists are still 'discovering' new muscles, including the Tensor Vastus Intermedius, located in the Quadriceps and recently 'found' in a new study. In my opinion this is contextual, dependent on what is being looked for whilst looking is going to influence what they find. Myers said, "While every anatomy text lists around 600 separate muscles, it is more accurate to say that there is one muscle poured into six hundred pockets of the fascial webbing."

This text will reference Flexibility Highways conceptualized by Chuck Wolf, which, in my opinion, is based more on the major muscles/tissue that control a motion rather than the depth or layer of their connections. The following descriptions of the Flexibility Highways are adapted from Chuck's descriptions and also found in his educational series.

Anterior Flexibility Highway

The anterior flexibility highway runs from the south to the north or along the sagittal plane with flexion/extension movements occurring on this highway. The muscles of this highway begin at the top the foot, moving up the leg and interchanges with the anterior compartment of the ankle and tibia and heads north through the patellar tendon through the knee and up into the quadriceps and hip flexors of the thigh. To enhance function of both the quadriceps and hip flexors, it is important to lengthen both together. The hip flexors of the thigh intersect with the abdominals of the lower trunk that travel to the ribs and progressing upward to the sternum where they venture into the pectorals of the chest, anterior shoulder, and the front of the neck. From there, an angular detour takes our journey into the jaw of the skull and up into the fascia of the scalp of the head. Following this concept, a case can be made that the range of motion in the southern section of the highway (that is, the lower leg) can affect the northern section (such as the trunk, chest, shoulder, neck or head). Further study of human motion enlightens us to analyze and understand the relationships that occur through chain reaction processes. The pictures below demonstrate the integrated stretching to enhance range of motion along the anterior aspect, or front of the body.

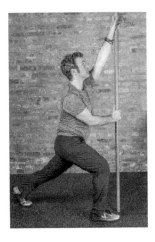 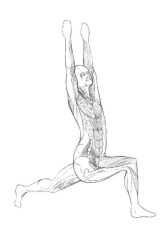 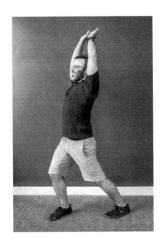

The anterior tissue of the body can be lengthened and strengthened together. This static motion can be progressed into an active motion via a lunge.

Posterior Flexibility Highway

The posterior flexibility highway runs from the south to the north, from the foot to the head, with flexion/extension movements occurring on this highway. The tissue of this highway begins on the bottom of the foot at the toe flexors and run through the posterior compartment of the ankle into the Achilles tendon. Continuing northward through the posterior calf group of the lower leg (Gastrocnemius, Soleus, and posterior tibialis), the knee interchange meets the hamstrings and takes the "hamstring expressway" into the ischial tuberosity of the pelvis, or what is affectionately called the sitting bones. These meet up with the gluteals and hamstrings and creates a multi-directional exchange north-by-northwest (or northeast depending upon which "leg" of the highway you travel) into the sacrolumbar junction. Now we're ready to move from the pelvis upward into the low back. Here the gluteals meet the erector spinae, in 'lumbar fascia junction', and head straight northward with many oblique interchanges of the spinal rotators along the way. The union of the gluteals and the erector spinae musculature of the back should be lengthened together in an integrated fashion because functional low back movement patterns includes the gluteals. Similar to the anterior highway, the final posterior journey terminates at the scalp fascia of the head. The pictures below demonstrate the integrated stretching to enhance range of motion along the posterior aspect of the body.

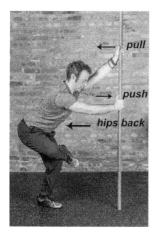 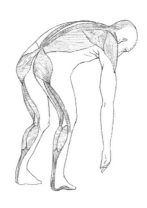 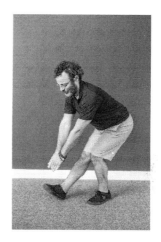

The posterior lines of the body can be lengthened and strengthened together, and can be progressed into an active motion via a lunge.

Lateral Flexibility Highway

A commonly overlooked pattern in movement is the lateral highway. The lateral flexibility highway runs from the south to the north along the side of the body from the foot and outside ankle all the way through the side ribs and finally terminating at the neck and head with abduction/adduction movements occurring on this highway. Running from the lateral ankle and the peroneal group the lateral highway goes north to the lateral tibial condyle near the knee and the iliotibial band of the thigh. Moving upward from this taut structure, the ITB merges with the tensor fascia lata in the upper part of the thigh, the gluteus medius and minimus within the pelvis, and meeting with the gluteus maximus, the most superficial muscle of the posterior pelvis. The gluteals are the "command central" of our center of gravity, balance, and power. They are utilized in all functional movement patterns, thus are the "hub" of tri-plane movement patterns. Along the lateral flexibility highway, the lateral gluteals are adjacent to the quadratus lumborum, which connects the pelvis with the lower ribs, and then the obliques. The obliques, running in a slight diagonal direction, merge with the external and internal intercostal muscles located between the ribs toward the anterior aspect and the latissimus dorsi located mainly in the lower back region but extending all the way to the upper arm in the posterior aspect of the body. From this point north, the lats will meet up with the posterior rotator cuff of the shoulder. Now here's an interesting point; a bypass occurs at the junction of the latissimus dorsi and the trapezius group, whereby the journey northbound moves through the trapezius group to the sternocleidomastoid of the neck. As the picture demonstrates, stretching the lateral highway is necessary for enhancement of frontal plane movement patterns such as running, swimming and swing sports, amongst others. For the optimal lateral stretch, think from the bottom up and let the hip move laterally off to the side as far as it can without undue strain.

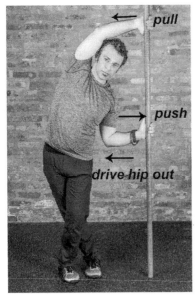 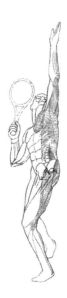

The lateral myofascial lines of the body can be stretched and strengthened together, and can be progressed into an active motion via a lateral lunge.

Anterior X & Posterior X Highway

When the anatomy and fiber alignment of the gluteals is viewed, it is interesting to note the near parallel and continuous fiber highway of the opposite latissimus dorsi and gluteus maximus. I call this the posterior X-factor, and for this reason try to stretch these muscle groups together. For instance, the tissue of the right latissimus dorsi and posteri shoulder sit on the same angle as the left gluteus complex, and when they lengthen together, work to decelerate the right arm when throwing. Another example is when a golfer takes their backswing; the opposite latissimus dorsi lengthens as well as the opposite gluteals. These muscles work in tandem to slow motion and therefore require to be stretched together in the cross-town highway, forming the X-Factor. For the anterior X-factor, I stretch the opposite hip flexor through the abdominals and obliques to the opposite shoulder. Therefore, I integrate those structures as these will be an enhancement for deceleration of functional movement patterns in the cross-body connections

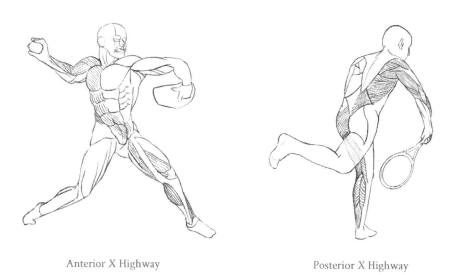

Anterior X Highway   Posterior X Highway

Additional Reading Suggestions:

Stecco, Luigi, John V. Basmanjian, and Julie Ann Day. Fascial Manipulation for Musculoskeletal Pain.

Myers, Thomas W. Anatomy Trains: Myofascial Meridians for Manual and Movement Therapists.

Wolf, Chuck. Flexibility Highways, www.humanmotionassociates.com

Brooks, Vernon B. The Neural Basis of Motor Control. New York: Oxford UP, 1986. Print.

Gray, Gary. Total body functional profile. Adrian, MI: Wynn Marketing.

Lindsay, Mark, and Chad Robertson. Fascia: Clinical Applications for Health and Human Performance.

Hammer, W. I. Functional soft tissue examination and treatment by manual methods: The extremities

Schliep, Robert. www.somatics.de

Earls, James. Born To Walk: Myofascial Efficiency and the Body in Movement.

3-Dimensional Movement Defined

Movement

Stevie Wonder is a favorite musician and recently took him off my list of people to see in concert before they die because I had the opportunity to see his Songs in the Key of Life tour. It was an amazing experience, and it was impressive how all the musicians worked together to create this beautiful, synchronous sound. Every instrument contributed its part to create the whole, and by synchronously playing arranged notes and chords, people were able to dance to some funky music. Movement, according to Merriam-Webster, is defined as being of "rhythmic character or quality, having a distinct structural unit and forming part of an extended (musical) composition." If looked at in the proper light, music and human movement share many qualities. Both need to be synchronous and have a rhythmic character or quality to be effective, and also have parts that form a larger composition. The joints of a dancer or gardener or anyone who moves are most efficient when there is synchrony and flow. Movement, relative to the body, is defined as "a sequencing of segments (Lenny Parracino, Functional Soft Tissue of the Hip, page 8).

In other words, motion needs to be a synchronous dissociation of body parts because if two bones move in the same speed in the same direction, the joint, defined as space between bones, doesn't feel any motion. Remember, bones move, joints feel, and muscles react to movement. This means that if movement is asynchronous there is going to be compensation in the system and won't look right. Dr. David Tiberio, PT, Ph.D., describes injury as occurring according to the Goldilocks principle, meaning too much motion, not enough motion, or motion at the wrong time.

KEY CONCEPT: Movement is a synchronous dissociation of body segments. If two bones move at the same speed and in the same direction, the joint doesn't feel. Think of Goldilocks: Too Much Motion; Not Enough Motion; Motion at the Wrong Time.

When someone is in pain, it's often evident by the way in which they move because they will move around a body part that hurts as opposed to through it. If the right hip is hurting or one is limited in the front of the hip, as they walk away (observed from the rear) often times you'd observe their right glut/pelvis come back towards you more during the extension phase vs the non-painful side.

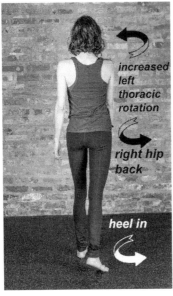 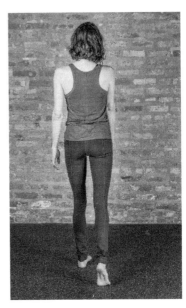

If a hip is limited into the second phase of gait, particularly extension, from a rear-view, it will appear as though the limited hip 'moves back' relative to the unaffected hip.

They demonstrate a "glitch in their hitch" of sorts. What's observed is somebody compensating by moving around as opposed to through their body part. This is important because it demonstrates an asymmetry in the movement system, and over time this will lead to further compensation. Even though the dysfunctional area hasn't yet been identified, asking WHY are the hips so asymmetrical can direct the course of the assessment.

In my experience, this is not the way the majority of movement professionals are taught, rather they target the pathologic tissue instead of what's above or below the site of the injury. This traditional lens of muscle function is one of isolation rather than integration, where the shortening (concentric) motion is described as the muscle action, and each muscle has an origin and insertion instead of an attachment.

For example, isolation describes the quadriceps as a knee extensor, with the origin (beginning) being the top of the femur and the insertion (end) being the patellar tendon into the tibia.

When these two points are brought together, the knee will extend, yet this is exactly the opposite of what the quadriceps do when working with other muscles and tissue to control the body as it reacts to the forces continuously presented to it, including gravity, ground forces, mass, and momentum. Through this integrated lens, in upright function it's seen that in the sagittal plane the quadriceps, in conjunction with other tissue, lengthens and controls knee flexion rather than extending the knee. When necessary, muscles CAN produce forces in order to create a motion; however acting upon anything requires a great deal of energy compared to REACTING to the environment in an integrated way that allows proper and efficient control.

> KEY CONCEPT: In integration, muscles lengthen to control forces presented to the body instead of shortening in isolation to produce a force.

To demonstrate the concept of muscles controlling forces rather than producing muscle contraction, place one hand overhead and one hand on your stomach. Take the overhead hand and reach backwards overhead (SEE PIC); what do you feel under the hand placed on your stomach? The answer should be tension, because the overhead hand reaching backwards lengthens the tissue under the hand (in this case the rectus abdominus, amongst others). The abdominal tissue didn't create any force; rather it was lengthened to control the momentum and mass of your hand reaching backwards. It was a subconscious reaction that simply happened, as opposed to a conscious contraction of your abdominals.

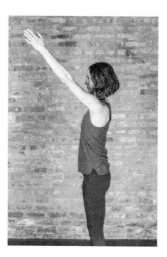

When the shoulder is flexed overhead, the abdominals lengthen to assist in controlling this motion.

Gravity, which constantly pulls down, and ground reaction forces work to counteract the pull of gravity, are opposing forces. As Sir Isaac Newton said, "Every action has an equal and opposite reaction," so the harder we hit the ground the harder the ground is going to push back up.

Mass and momentum must also be appreciated within the equation of truths that influence movement. Mass is the quantity of matter that a body contains, as measured by its acceleration under force, or by the force exerted on it by a gravitational field. Momentum is the quantity of motion of a moving body, measured as a product of its mass and velocity.

For example, if a ball is rolled down a hill, it will continue to gain momentum until it encounters another force that will slow it down, such as another hill. According to Ida Rolf, people work with or fight against gravity while staying upright. Those working against gravity tend to demonstrate a less than ideal posture, often including a forward head and rounded upper back. This position is strongly correlated with sitting and working at a computer, and has increased with the advancement of technology and sedentary lifestyles. It's proven that for every inch of forward head posture, the weight of the head on the spine increases by an additional 10 pounds (Kapandji, 2008). Forward head posture is associated with headaches, decreased range of motion, loss of lung capacity, and other postural and emotional changes. Improved and 'tall' posture facilitates the free flow of digestion, metabolism, and elimination, and it also improves the ability of the body to dissociate segments of a larger whole, in order to accomplish an intended task. Remember, movement is defined as a sequential dissociation of segments.

KEY CONCEPT: Human Movement—defined as a sequential dissociation of body segments.

Real and Relative Motion

Most often, injury occurs when forces are presented that the body can't handle, unless it's a crush injury. Injury typically occurs when the body should transition the force load into the unload/utilization of forces, a point in time the Gray Institute calls the Transformational Zone (TZ). Within this paradigm, the quadriceps will control sagittal plane knee flexion while also controlling frontal and transverse plane motion. This is opposite of the isolated action taught in books, where the muscles on the front of the thigh create knee extension.

While muscles CAN create force, they're more efficient and effective while controlling and reacting to the external forces presented to them by taking advantage of the internal tensile forces that are transmitted from one part to another. Within this framework it's also more challenging to comprehend that when the foot hits the ground at the first TZ of gait, the quadriceps control frontal plane abduction and transverse plane internal rotation in addition to flexion, along with tissue above and below the knee.

The concept of tissue lengthening first in order to control gravity, ground reaction, mass and momentum fits into other systems and enhances the mindset and paradigm of treatment options within any given practice. Injury typically occurs at the TZ, and if the Transformational Zone for a particular activity is known, then assessing if the joint feels the triplane motion can be checked. If the joint isn't feeling a specific motion in a specific plane, then this paradigm let's WHY be asked and answered logically and effectively.

KEY CONCEPT:

Injury occurs when forces are presented to the body that the body cannot handle at the end of the transformational zone.

Every action has at least two transformational zones.

Transformational Zone (TZ) is defined as the point in time when the body stops loading and begins to unload.

Motor control theories, including facilitatory and inhibitory techniques, and sequential firing patterns of muscles are better comprehended with the understanding that if muscles can't lengthen, or go opposite first, then proprioceptors aren't fully stimulated, potentially contributing to inhibitions. Vernon Brooks stated that "When the tone of opposing muscles is unequal, one muscle shortens and the other is stretched, rotating the joint to a new angle where their tensions are equal." Often times muscles are inhibited because the length tension relationship of a joint is altered, and the surrounding tissue then can't efficiently control forces and results in altered sequential firing patterns at the Motor Control Center (MCC).

Examples of isolated muscle function, or what can be called a "7 Ocean Mentality of Movement", can be found in any number of books. The 7 Ocean mentality, like isolated muscle, is a manmade construct because if the quad is looked at in isolation, or as 1 of the 7 oceans, it extends the knee. Yet this is merely part of the equation because the quadriceps prefers to work in conjunction with other tissue to control motion that it reacts to. Like all muscles in the body, it can work in isolation in order to create a motion at a joint, but in this paradigm, a muscle 'creates' a force first by shortening, rather than 'controls' a force by first lengthening.

Proprioception is defined as an awareness of self in space, and proprioceptors are found in soft tissue including fascia and particularly joint capsules. Proprioceptors must first lengthen, which creates an environment that will authentically stimulate the nervous system and allow neuroplastic changes to movement patterning that can change the way a movement is accomplished. It was once thought that proprioceptors were only found in joints and joint capsules, however recent research has demonstrated that proprioceptors are readily found in the fascia, and that proprioceptors in the joints are only active at end range motions.

Movement is three dimensional, asymmetrical, and spiral in nature rather than linear and symmetrical, and can be seen as a synchronous dissociation of body segments. Asymmetries are evidenced throughout the body, setting up for functional asymmetries too. These asymmetries include 3 left lung lobes and 2 on the right, one liver, one spleen and the asymmetrical connections of the hip flexors into the diaphragm. The result is inherent asymmetry and the uneven distribution of forces throughout the system. Similar to a helix, when gravity pulls our bodies down it doesn't purely compress; rather, it escapes through rotation and causes a combination of alternating compressive and tensile forces.

Through myofascial release (such as foam rolling and manual therapy) and appropriate movement, working towards greater symmetry is the objective. The transmission of tension through tensegrity structures allows for a distribution of forces to all interconnected elements. It also couples the whole system mechanically as one, rather than forcing one part to accept all the forces presented. This model allows for the entire system to distribute the forces simultaneously.

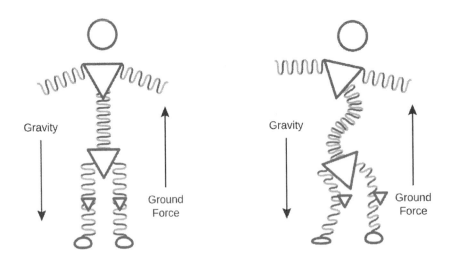

The body is a helical structure, and gravity doesn't compress a helical structure, rather it escapes through rotation. When there is asymmetry in the body, which there is in everyone based on anatomy, the body rotates around a vertical axis, tensioning some areas and compressing other in 3 planes of motion.

This compression/tension relationship can occur at a joint, where one side is compressed and the other side is more tensioned, or due to the three dimensionality of the body can occur with compression above and below and tension in the middle. This allows for stability and mobility at each segment. As a structure sways, the (fascial) tensegrity network stretches in the middle and compresses above and below, also aligned with the joint by joint approach popularized by Gray Cook. This can be felt in the body when standing tall and reaching for something. What is felt is a stretch in the middle of the body (or core), and compression (or muscle engagement) above and below, or vice versa.

Concurrently, when looked at three dimensionally, the spine and vertebrae also feel compression on one side and tension on the other while reaching.

Describing motion at a joint

In order to create an environment unique to the patient, a thorough understanding of the specific movements unique to INDIVIDUAL is paramount. If we know what they want to accomplish, a 3D movement assessment that replicates the specific task can be performed in order to see if what should happens does, which is analyzed at the Transformational Zones (TZ). When a region of the body is restricted and unable to fully lengthen and dissociate, it often moves at the same speed as the bone above/below, resulting in no dissociation (or relative movement) of one bone against another. One bone must move faster or slower than the bone above/below for proprioceptors to lengthen and be stimulated, movement needs to be a synchronous dissociation of body parts. If one part moves in the same speed in the same direction, proprioceptors won't lengthen, and therefore the joint won't FEEL any motion.

There are few studies or books about relative motions, or how one body part must move faster or slower than the part above/below for relative motion to be felt. However in the book Visceral Manipulation, by Jean Pierre Barral, the author does briefly refer to relative motions while discussing how one organ past another. "If a subject stands and bends forward at the waist, his liver will move forward, sliding over the duodenum and the hepatic flexure of the colon below. The liver and the hepatic flexure will both move inferiorly, but the liver more so, since it moves first and farthest with flexion. Thus we can say that the liver slides antero-inferiorly over the duodenum and hepatic flexure, even if these other structures move in the same direction. Similar processes occurs in the other viscera (page 4). This passage accurately reflects that depending on how much motion is driven to a specific part, surfaces are going to move further and faster than what is above or below. The body is INTERRELATED and REACTS to gravity, ground reaction forces, mass and momentum, rather than 658 different muscles acting independently.

When assessing movement, considering joint motion and how one bone plays against another is the primary objective. In order to describe joint motion, it is helpful to follow a consistent thought process, namely bones move, joints feel, and muscles react to movement. If two bones move in the same speed at the same direction, then the joint doesn't feel anything because movement is a synchronous dissociation of body segments.

KEY CONCEPT: If two bones move at the same speed in the same direction, the resultant joint motion is zero.

Describing Relative Joint Motion

Joint: space between bones

1) What 2 bones make up the joint?

2) Are bones moving in same or opposite direction in each plane?

3) Top faster than bottom? Bottom faster than top?

The Five ways a joint can feel the same motion

Remember that in the extremities, motion is named for how a distal bone moves on a fixed proximal bone. Yet, there are few times when one bone moves and another stays still. Instead bone bones move in the same or opposite direction, with one moving faster or slower than the one above or below. This is analogous to one train moving right out of the other trains window. For this to happen, one train has to move faster or slower than the other so that, from Train A's perspective, Train B is moving to the right.

The following pictures describe the combinations of movement that can result in train B moving out of Train A's window to the right. As an analogy, Train A is the tibia, or distal bone, and Train B is the femur, or proximal bone, and the space between the two trains/bones is the 'knee joint'.

Recall that bones move, joints feel or sense the bone movement, and muscles react to the forces that create the bone motion; and if bones move in the same direction at the same speed, despite the bone motion, the joint won't sense any motion. If both trains move in the same direction at the same speed, Train B will never move out of train A's window to the right.

In picture 1, the distal bone stays still and the proximal bone moves right.

In picture 2, the distal bone moves left on a fixed proximal, still resulting in Train B moving right from train A's perspective.

In picture 3, the distal bone moves one direction and the proximal bone moves in the opposite direction, resulting in Train B moving right from Train A's perspective.

In picture 4, the distal bone moves in the direction, and the proximal bone moves in the direction faster, resulting in Train B moving to the right from Train A's perspective.

In picture 5, Train A moves to the left faster than Train B. Both bones move in the same direction with the distal bone moving faster than the proximal, resulting in train B moving right from Train A's perspective.

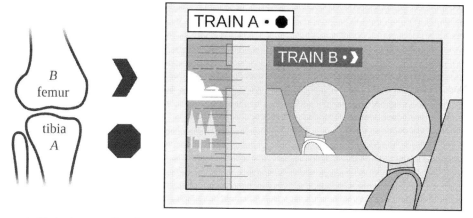

Picture 1. Train A stays still and train B moves to the right, resulting in Train B moving out of Train A's window to the right.

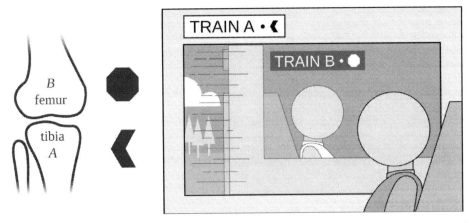

Picture 2. Train A moves to the left, and Train B stays still, resulting in Train B moving out of Train A's window to the right.

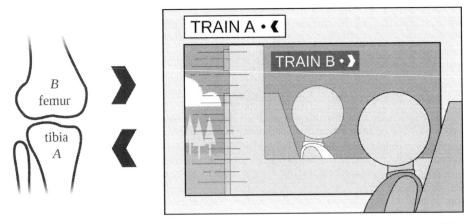

Picture 3. Train A moves to the left and train B moves to the right, resulting in Train B moving out of Train A's window to the right.

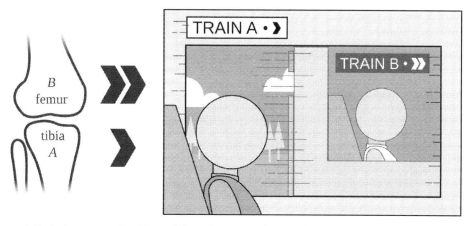

Picture 4. Train A moves to the right, and Train B moves to the right faster than train A, resulting in Train B moving out of Train A's window to the right.

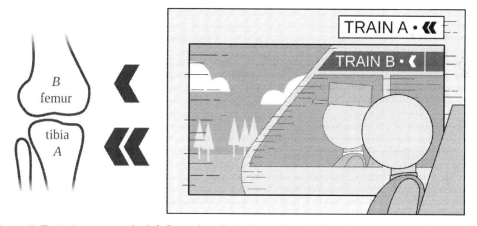

Picture 5. Train A moves to the left faster than Train B, resulting in Train B moving out of Train A's window to the right.

Drivers

A driver is a way to create a reaction, and according to the Gray Institute, relative to naming joint motion, a driver is defined as using a body part to subconsciously create motion into another body part.

When both bones move in the same direction with the top moving faster, it implies a top down driver. A top down driver implies that motion comes from above and that the top bone moves further and faster in the direction of movement, relative to the bottom bone. When bones move in the same direction with the bottom moving faster, it implies a bottom up driver because the bottom bone moves faster in a direction.

Top-Down vs. Bottom-Up

Top-Down Driver: Proximal bones move in a direction faster than the distal bones

Bottom-Up Driver: Distal bones move in a direction faster than the proximal bones.

A Driver is a way to create a reaction

For example, while standing with feet shoulder width apart and eyes forward, when the left hand is rotated left at shoulder height, or behind the body, if the eyes remain forward the body feels right cervical rotation. In this instance, the left arm is considered a bottom up driver into the cervical spine. If the head remains focused forward, the cervical spine experiences right rotation, even though most of the bones of the cervical spine will be rotating left in space. Even though the bones are moving left in space because they react to the bottom bones moving, because the bottom bones move left faster than the top bones, and because of how motion is named in the spine, the cervical spine feels right rotation. Left cervical segment rotation is considered the real bone motion, while right cervical rotation is considered the relative joint motions. Concurrently, that same left arm is a top down driver into the joints below causing right foot pronation and left foot supination via a chain reaction.

The front leg in gait reacts to a bottom up driver because upon heel strike, ground forces are lateral to the center of the subtalar joint, creating a calcaneal eversion moment, and allowing the talus to fall down and in towards middle upon heel strike. This talus motion creates motion down into the forefoot and up into the tibia and joints above.

This happens because the center of gravity is medial to the calcaneus, forcing the tibia to rotate inward towards midline, but not as far or as fast as the talus. Through this reaction, transverse plane tibial rotation should create femur rotation in the same direction, but not as far or as fast as the tibia. For example, when the left foot hits the ground, the left calcaneus everts for free, causing the talus to drop in towards middle. The talar motion towards midline causes the left tibia to rotate right towards middle, but not as far or as fast as the talus. The chain reaction forces the femur to follow in towards midline, also rotating right, however not as far or as fast as the tibia below.

All of this motion is given to the system for free that the body has to control, and if one part isn't able to coordinate and synchronize movement effectively, the result is too much motion somewhere to compensate for what isn't doing enough. The part that is doing too much often is the sight of the injury, or the victim, while the criminal remains silent.

For example, while analyzing transverse triplane motion of the knee at the point in time when the foot hits the ground, or for any joint at any time, following a systematic thought process is helpful. The first step is defining what two bones make up the joint being assessed. Recall that a joint is space between bones, and attempting to understand the 3D relationship of what one bone is doing against another is the objective. Relative to the knee, the two bones are the tibia and femur because the patella is along for the ride following the tibia and femur.

At heel strike, because of ground reaction forces and the joints relation to midline, the calcaneus everts (for free) and causes the talus to adduct towards midline. This forces tibial inward rotation, slower than the talus below, causing the femur to follow suit, but not as far or as fast as what is below. This reaction continues, where bones move in the same direction with the bottom bone moving faster until dissipated somewhere around the TL junction, depending on individual structure.

The second rule to identify 3D joint motion is to distinguish whether bones move in the same or opposite direction in each plane, relative to the intended task. For example, in gait, when the right foot hits the ground the right tibia rotates internally, responds to the talus adducting as a result of calcaneal eversion. Motion is driven from the bottom when the foot hits the ground, and the right femur internally rotates following the tibia inward, but not as far or as fast. When the bones making up the joint move in the same direction, the third rule to identify 3D joint motion must be considered, which is to understand which bone is moving faster, the top or the bottom.

Understanding that at heel strike, the tibia should internally rotate/move towards middle at a faster rate than the femur is critical. Quite often I have found that those with patellofemoral knee pain, particularly at heel strike with running, jumping, lunging, walking, or stairs, is because the tibia doesn't rotate inwards faster than the femur at the first TZ. This results in the patella smacking into the lateral femoral condyle and upsetting all the 'stuff' on the anterior-lateral side of the knee. Traditionally we would blame the VMO (inside quad muscles) for not working properly; however looking through the lens of integrated movement we can see that it's not typically the VMO's fault.

KEY CONCEPT: When the foot hits the ground, the tibia should move in the direction faster than the femur, because in the transverse plane the tibia should move inward.

Recall that in the extremities, motion is named for the distal bone moving on a fixed proximal bone, yet this infrequently happens because most times when one bone moves and the other remains fixed. Rather, they either move in the same or opposite direction, and if moving in the same direction most often one bone is moving faster than the other. Therefore, understanding what SHOULD happen is imperative, because the bones could be moving in one direction and the joint could be FEELING exactly the opposite, which is why the 3rd rule (which bone moves faster, the top or bottom) is important. In this instance, when the foot hits the ground at heel strike, because it's a bottom up driver, the knee should FEEL internal rotation, because the tibia is moving towards middle faster than femur. At least it SHOULD, and if it doesn't the question WHY must be asked.

1st Transformational Zone

	Sagittal	Frontal	Transverse
Hip	Flexion	ADduction	Internal Rotation
Knee	Flexion	ABduction	Internal Rotation
Ankle	PF/DF		ABD/ADD
Subtalar		Eversion	ABduction
MidTarsal	DF	Inversion	ABDuction

This graph demonstrates the triplane motion of the lower extremity when the foot hits the ground.

Back Leg: Driven from the Top Down in Gait

While the front foot is a bottom up driver into the system, the trail leg experiences a top down motion, with some exceptions. When the right leg becomes the back leg during left leg swing phase, momentum of the left foot swinging forward causes the pelvis to rotate right. This causes the right femur to also rotate right, but not as far or fast as the pelvis. Right femur rotation causes the tibia to also rotate right, forcing the talus to climb back atop the calcaneus in response to tibial motion. This chain reaction creates calcaneal inversion and the resultant locking of the midfoot required for propulsion at toe off.

During gait, even though the right femur and right tibia bones are rotating right, or externally in space at the second TZ, the knee should feel relative internal rotation. Tradition has taught that the knee externally rotates at the second phase of gait however, it actually feels MORE internal rotation. This is because motion in the extremities is named for how the distal bone moves on a fixed proximal bone. Recall that bones move, joints feel and muscles react, and if two bones move in the same direction (real bone external rotation), more than likely one bone will be moving faster. In this situation, the top bone moves faster because it is driven from the opposite leg swinging forward in preparation for heel strike. Therefore, following the rule of naming motion in an extremity, the distal moves on a fixed proximal and the joint feels internal rotation. Even though both bones are rotating externally in space, the knee feels internal rotation because of how motion in extremities is named. Knee external rotation is felt during swing phase up until the heel hits the ground when the entire process starts over.

KEY CONCEPT: Motion in the extremities is named for the distal bone moving on a fixed proximal bone. In the spine motion is named for the proximal bone moving on a fixed distal.

This matters because it's important to create as proprioceptively realistic environment as possible and is applicable for the person experiencing knee pain, especially at the first phase of gait. Often the knee feels an external rotation moment when it should feel internal rotation. When this happens, the tibia moves externally faster than the femur, creating asynchrony in the system and a situation where the patella smack into the lateral condyle of the femur. It's not the VMO's fault that the patella tracked laterally, rather the lack of timing of the femur moving externally relative to the tibia. If the three steps to assessing joint motion are followed, understanding relative joint motion and that the knee feels internal rotation becomes easier to assess.

If you know what should happen at a joint, then seeing if it happens or not is easier, and if not you must ask WHY. The dysfunction is probably in the foot or hip, and when the limited joint mobility is increased, then the joints above or below won't have to make up the difference in motion.

For example, knee motion at the second TZ:

What two bones? Tibia and femur

Same direction or opposite direction? Same direction because motion is being driven from the opposite leg swinging forward in space.

Which bone is moving faster, the top or bottom? Top is moving faster in the direction because it's being driven from the opposite leg swinging forward.

Therefore the knee feels internal rotation because both bones are moving in the same direction but the top is moving faster than the bottom.

KEY CONCEPT:

Understanding the reason why someone is having pain or dysfunction can be difficult. While we all strive to answer that question as best as we can, often times there are circumstances beyond what we are able to help with.

Therefore, as a clinician, having other medical professionals on your team is important. We are not islands unto ourselves, and so we should have clinicians from various other medical professions on our 'Team', including 1-2 non-surgical physicians, 1-2 surgeons, chiropractor/osteopath, physical therapist, massage therapist, podiatrist (or someone to make orthotics) and 1-2 personal trainers.

In addition, an understanding of current pain science is helpful. This topic has purposefully not been addressed much in this text. Not being able to effectively answer "why" is a huge driver for me personally to continue to learn and expand as a person and clinician.

Additional Reading Suggestions

Gray, G. Functional Video Digest Series. Vol 3.4 Functional Manual Reaction- The Foot and Ankle, Vol. 3.8 Proprioceptors.

Rolf, Ida P., and Rosemary Feitis. Rolfing and Physical Reality

Vernon Brooks: The Neural Basis for Motor Control

Cook, G. Movement Functional Movement Systems: Screening, Assessment, Corrective Strategies

Barral, J. P., and Pierre Mercier. Visceral Manipulation.

Gambetta, Vern. www.functionalpathtrainingblog.com

CHAPTER 4

Motor Control Theories and Their Importance in 3D Movement

As mentioned, the body continually reacts to its environment and surroundings, and the brain is responsible for coordinating and synchronizing the actions and reactions of muscles, in reconciling the afferent input from the environment. Movement is governed in regions of the cerebral cortex, particularly in the Motor Cortex and also the Motor Control Center (MCC) located in the cerebellum. The motor cortex receives instructions from the association cortex, the cerebellum, and the basal ganglia, and issues commands to the spinal cord, and are connected through various feedback loops for messages going up and down. The motor cortex operates at a lower level than the cerebral cortex, and assists in how to carry out movements for a given strategy (Brooks). The brain continually is receiving input from the periphery, and dysfunction arises when there is aberrant afferent input into the MCC. This creates compensatory patterns of muscles and their ability to fire in a proper and sequential order. This can cause a pattern of facilitations leading to inhibitions, which can perpetuate the negative feedback loop. Through my learnings and studies with people smarter than I, I now believe that really what we are doing is altering the aberrant afferent input in order to change the output firing pattern.

In his book The Neural Basis for Motor Control, Vernon Brooks discusses the hierarchy of motor control, and the following is an example of the process. Let's say I want to open the bottom drawer of my dresser to get my favorite t-shirt. Before I reach down to get it, many things are required in a sequenced chain of command. First the limbic system demands that I "fill my needs" before the cerebral cortex selects a strategy. "Go this way". After that, the motor control center (MCC), where says, "Get your shirt this way now", onto the spine that says "do it" before this neural information arrives at the muscles, where "doing it" is done.

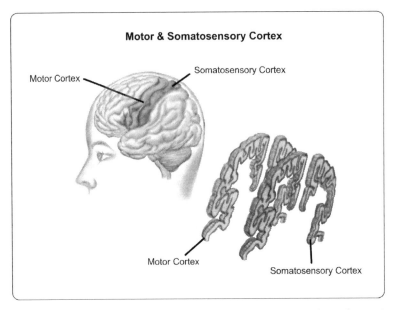

Motor & Somatosensory Cortex

Motor Cortex

Somatosensory Cortex

Motor Cortex

Somatosensory Cortex

Sensory input into the brain is translated into motor output. Chronic pain results in changes in the representation of the painful body part, what Lorimer Mosely refers to as "smudging". Part of any rehabilitation program must incorporate creating more representation in the brain.

Through many attempts and failures while learning a new task, the baby finally achieves success. This is secondary to the MCC coordinating the movement and "learning" how to do it correctly, until happening without "thinking". After an injury or an aberrant movement pattern, compensation occurs and the MCC adapts to this compensation pattern. Often this results in holding that pattern, altering the sequential firing through the movement and, unless changed, will become further engrained in a movement and ultimately part of the permanent pattern; for example, a whiplash accident where the posterior muscles brace for the anterior neck muscles, where the posterior neck becomes tight and painful, regardless of massage, stretching and strengthening. Until and unless the aberrant afferent input into the MCC is altered, the pattern will remain. There are many tools that attempt to alter this neurological relationship, including Applied Kinesiology, Clinical Kinesiology and Proprioceptive Deep Tendon Reflex (PDT-R) (the second two are offshoots of Applied Kinesiology) among many others. I believe the tool that should be used is the one the practitioner is comfortable with, and allows the most insight into the nervous system. Remember, all we are trying to do is alter the perception with the nervous system and the aberrant afferent input in, in order to make the nervous system more efficient, increase function and decrease pain. This is accomplished through a multi-faceted approach.

Reciprocal inhibition can be defined as a neuromuscular reflex, where an increased neural drive of a muscle or group of muscles reduces the neural activity of functional antagonists. It is not a simple function of "on or off", as postural dysfunction resulting in adaptive shortening and hypertonicity inhibits functional antagonists, such as an upregulated or facilitated piriformis that could potentially inhibit the psoas. The piriformis does not decrease the neural drive to the psoas completely, as it's possible to move and function, just less than optimally. What this means is that merely stretching or strengthening a muscle isn't enough because it doesn't reprogram the MCC. The first objective becomes WHEN does the muscle need to be used and for what purpose? The second objective is then to create the environment that resequences the system, first by down regulating the up regulated tissue and then up regulating the down regulated tissue, which most times are paired. The trick, however, is how to know what tissues are paired in a facilitation and inhibition, which can be accomplished by following a thought process. There are many "systems" of muscle testing, including Neurokinetic Therapy (NKT), which is the discipline I utilize the most.

According to Vernon Brooks in the article "Motor Control How Posture and Movement are Governed":

"Strong reciprocal inhibition allows the limb to swing loose, that is, to be compliant. Joints are made more compliant before the onset of a planned movement. Weak reciprocal inhibition, in contrast, permits co-contraction of opposing muscles, which makes the joint stiff. The golfer holds his arms fairly stiff during the hold before the swing, but they are compliant during the swing and then stiffen again before the impact. Therapists can increase or decrease unwanted actions through appropriate touch, pressure, or imposed postures. Repetition of these movements and understanding of what is wanted by the patient can help involve larger task systems and can thus build new, voluntary capabilities on the initial changes produced by the therapist".

KEY CONCEPT: A simplified example of reciprocal inhibition is the nervous system sending a message to a muscle to contract, creating tension in the opposing muscle on the other side of the joint, and inhibiting (decreasing the impulse from the motor neurons) in order for the joint to move. Sometimes, there are aberrant, afferent inputs, which results in altered efferent motor output. In crude terms, if a muscle is too connected to the nervous system, it will "steal" the juice from other muscles ability to contract, and therefore the motor output will also be altered. This happens often with pain. From a 'muscle testing' perspective, this can be looked at as 'facilitated' or 'inhibited' tissue. Please note that the term 'inhibited', does not mean that a muscle is not "working", or not connected to the system. Rather the timing and ability of the nervous system to engage the tissue is decreased, resulting in a delayed and often times weakened muscle contraction. Sometimes these facilitation to inhibition relationships can be from one side of the joint to the other, and many other times these relationships are elsewhere, sometimes close, and other times farther away. My friend and teacher of NKT, Thomas Wells, advises starting within 18 inches of the injury and work your way out. Clinically, I've found that often times, the facilitation to inhibition relations lies on the same myofascial line, for whatever combination of tissue would have to control the dysfunctional/painful movement.

Ensuring each joint (defined as a space between bones) moves independently from the other joints in any given movement is imperative. The concept of a joint needing independency before interdependency works well within the context of one bone needing to move at a different speed than the bone above or below for a synchronous dissociation of parts to occur. If two bones move in the same speed in the same direction the joint doesn't feel anything, resulting in interdependent movement between joints.

If there is a pinch on the closing angle side of a joint, Dr. Andreo Spina, DC, creator of Functional Range Conditioning (FRC), a fantastic approach to the body that stresses joint independence before joint interdependence, says it's indicative of an unhealthy joint and needs to be addressed before clearing the surrounding soft tissue. Pinching points in the closing angle of an articular motion means there is joint dysfunction. During a joint's full articular rotation, the sensation should be on the opening side of the joint, not the closing side, and if not there is either a neurological or structural limitation (or both). If it is on the opening side of the joint it's typically a tissue extensibility problem and should be worked into and through. However, with a closing angle pinch the joint mobility must be resolved first, prior to addressing tissue dysfunction.

When working with a compressed and/or impinged joint, recognizing that a compressed joint and a joint that provides an aberrant response to compression are not the same thing, although often they're found together. Because of this, and based on the principle of reciprocal inhibition, differentially diagnosing why a joint is stiff becomes important, because often times the nervous system will compress a joint to offer stability to an otherwise unstable system. What this means is that depending on WHY it is compressed, mobilizing the joint may or may not be the best course of action. For example, sometimes people that have an anterior hip impingement have muscles that test weak and upon distraction the muscles test strong, while other times muscles test weak upon distraction and strong upon compression. If someone experiences hip impingement and they test strong upon compression and weak with distraction, I wouldn't distract the hip, rather provide exercises to strengthen the hip. Conversely, the hip that is impinged that has muscles that get strong with distraction would receive a treatment that involved hip distraction followed by strengthening. (See differential diagnosis section for more discussion).

KEY CONCEPT: Addressing closing angle joint restrictions is a priority before addressing soft tissue restriction.

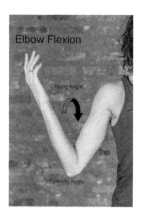 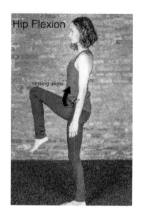 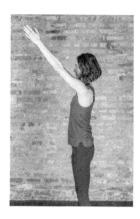

Closing angle binding is often indicative of capsular restrictions and should be addressed first.

Case Example: Mary

Mary is a grandmother of 2 who has neck pain. She was heading to her daughter's Christmas party when her car slid on black ice and she ended up the middle car in a three car pile-up, getting hit in the passenger side rear first before hitting the car in front of her. Thankfully, she wasn't majorly hurt; however, she did sustain a whiplash accident and needed physical and manual therapy, which helped to a point but never fully resolved, despite 2 separate episodes of therapy with other clinicians. When I met Mary, her posterior muscles were bracing for the anterior neck muscles, and she demonstrated significant restrictions with neck flexion, side bending and rotating bilaterally, with difficulty into left rotation and side bending more than right. She was miserable physically and also emotionally because her dysfunction was affecting all aspects of her life. She was waking up at least 1-2 times per night because of pain, and also was unable to participate in her leisure time activities including tennis.

Mary demonstrated limited postural awareness, forward head, increased thoracic kyphosis and rounded shoulders, in addition to being a chest breather, using her accessory muscles for respiration. The anxiety about the situation was evident, and she was discouraged about her situation, frustrated with the lack of ability to make physical changes and motivated to do what it took to get her life back to normal.

Because Mary had been other places seeking to resolve her issues, I decided to take an approach that was less on "increasing motion" and more about stimulating her parasympathetic nervous system, recognizing that she will be able to respond more to changes in her MCC if she is less anxious and stimulated.

I felt she was stuck in a negative feedback loop, something common to people in pain and experiencing dysfunction. Because it hurts to move, she holds tight and braces to protect, tightening tissues, and making flow of blood and lymph through tissue more difficult. In addition, her anxious behavior including shallow chest breaths and her guarding and pain with movement caused her to body to be in "protect and defend mode", or in a sympathetic state. Her anxiety caused tightness and more stimulation, making it difficult to breathe and move freely, causing more anxiety. In addition, her posture altered the length tension relationship of her joints and tissue, lengthening the neck flexors and shortening the extensors. This often times leads to altered connection to the nervous system, where the shortened tissue, in this case the extensors, are more connected than the lengthened tissue on the other side of the joint.

We began our session with some simple breathing and mindfulness exercises, including diaphragmatic breaths with long, slow exhales. We also discussed the process which occurs in her body with in a sympathetic nervous system state, including anxiety, shallow breaths, and being on guard. Our first session also consisted of proprioceptive exercises to make her aware of where she carries herself in space, particularly with the alignment of her head relative to her shoulders and hips. She was educated on the importance of first down-regulating her nervous system in order to then reprogram the painful movement pattern that she found herself in. Professionally, I've found that simply being educated on this process, including slow and mindful breathing and a 'reversal of posture exercise', is a very powerful first step in treatment, rather than me "doing something" via manual therapy. By the end of the first session, her pain from 8/10 to 5/10, with an increased ability to rotate her neck; but more importantly a positive outlook and mental attitude about the direction of treatment and that she WILL get better.

In our second session she was responsive enough to figure out that her suboccipital muscles were working hard, resulting in less neural drive to the neck flexors and cervical rotators. This fits into her description of leading with her head and also having these muscles assist in respiration. After her second session, there was a reduction of pain to 3/10 and demonstrated even more cervical ROM. Simply by re-programming the movement at her motor control center, combined with a positive outlook on her situation and providing her awareness of her dysfunction, by the 6th session she was pain free and back to playing tennis, as well as sleeping through the night.

Mary's sessions with me were beneficial where other sessions hadn't been because we dealt with her nervous system first. Through promoting a parasympathetic response, combined with breathing, releasing, and activating the correct combination of tissue and altering her mindset, we were able to reprogram her movement and give her the tools to keep herself out of pain. It also demonstrates the importance of tying the appropriate combination of dysfunctional muscles together to create change. Other episodes of therapy had failed because her dysfunction was looked at from a pure musculoskeletal perspective rather than from a holistic perspective where the hierarchy of needs puts survival and stability of the system before mobility. By working to create a parasympathetic response, a feed forward loop was created where her ability to relax and breathe from her diaphragm lessened her anxiety and sympathetic response, allowing a musculoskeletal change to her system.

Additional Reading

Vernon Brooks: The Neural Basis for Motor Control

Brooks VB: Motor Control How posture and movement are governed.

Feldenkrais, M., & Beringer, E. (2010). Embodied wisdom: The collected papers of Moshe´ Feldenkrais.

Weinstock, David. NeuroKinetic Therapy: An Innovative Approach to Manual Muscle Testing

Rosen, Richard. The Yoga of Breath, A Step by Step Guide to Pranayama

CHAPTER 5

Integration of Fascia & Nervous System

From conception we develop and grow with slight variations in structural arrangement and development because we don't all start from the same blank slate, as structure will biomechanically be slightly different from one to another. Vern Inman said "A conclusion that seems inescapable is that each of us learns to integrate the numerous variables that nature has bestowed upon our individual neuromusculoskeletal systems into a smoothly functioning whole" (Science in the Art of Osteopathy, p98). I like this quote because we are a summation of our experiences and thoughts up to this present time, not to mention the asymmetrical organs and muscle attachments. Nature and nurture both influence the people we are, and with this understanding I have become a much better clinician.

Tensegrity

The concept of tensegrity was popularized in 1961 by engineer Buckminster Fuller. Tensegrity is the property certain structures possess of maintaining their integrity as a result of continuous tensile integrity, rather than continuous compressive integrity (Pienta & Coffey, 1991).

Tensegrity-based structures are composed of a series of continuous tension resistant components, such as myofascia, and a discontinuous series of compression resistant elements, such as bones, and describe structures that stabilize themselves mechanically by balancing local compression with continuous tension

Tensegrity structures are pre-stressed and require continuous transmission of internal tensions to maintain stability, analogous to the resting tone the central nervous system (CNS) keeps in muscle.

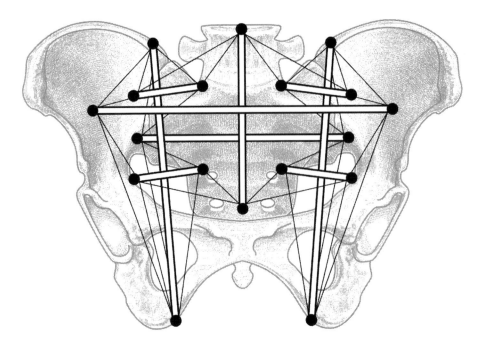

Tensegrity, or tension within integrity, describes how myofascia is a series of continuous tension resistant components and a discontinuous series of compression resistant elements. This means that with tension comes compression, and with compression comes tension.

The Adaptable Fascia

Fascia responds to mechanical interventions by changing the volume and consistency of ground substance, while decreasing the cross linked fibers developed as a result of the inflammatory process. The main goal is to increase the inter-fiber distance so that compression is reduced and increased extensibility of tissue is achieved (Scarr, *Biotensegrity: the structural basis of life*, 2014).

This process happens in daily life through repetitive stress or strain to a region of the body. The inherent asymmetry in the body results in asymmetrical distribution of forces that result in gravity pulling our helical bodies into a further asymmetrical position.

The result is some tissue becomes longer, and over time pain develops as a result of tissue being restricted and immobile. The importance of bodywork, whether self or otherwise, is the reintroduction of movement and separations of the different layers of the tissue. This is accomplished by pushing fluids around the body, allowing blood and oxygen to get to the tissue. Bodywork increases flow, allows fluid and space between tissues to be preserved and promotes flow, and this feeds forward into a more positive movement, promoting even more flow.

As a result of soft tissue injury, the ability of tissue to slide and glide past each other becomes limited, leading to stagnant fluid in the tissue. This can lead to a solidification of the layers of fascia against each other. As a manual therapist, it is something that can be felt as an abrupt tensioning of `tissue in one area and is often uncomfortable for the client.

> KEY CONCEPT: The ability of tissue to slide and glide past each other is important and, if limited, often can be felt as increased and abrupt tension in a specific region.

Once the inflammation cycle begins, and after a tissue is injured, the tissue starts to fibrose the injured area in an effort to repair the tissue. This fibrotic and remodeled connective tissue is lower in tensile strength and stiffer than normal tissue secondary to randomized collagen fiber direction, and the inability of the collagen bundles to slide easily over one another. This is due to the cross linking fibers and lack of hydration, and because the substituted collagen types aren't as strong as the original. However, this strategy doesn't take into account the role of the CNS in mitigating extensibility and tone of tissue.

When the body experiences pain during soft tissue release (self or otherwise), the CNS via somatovisceral and somato-parasympathetic reflexes releases neurotransmitters and increases the parasympathetic nervous system, allowing relaxed breathing and less hypertonic tissue. Another way to say that is when the body experiences painful stimulus from the nervous system reflex, the body releases transmitters that increase the ability to "rest and digest" and release the tissue that's being held tight by the nervous system. This potentially could be why people describe a sense of lightness and free-ness in the tissue after a release, and could be a 'window' to the nervous system that is necessary to reinforce changes in the nervous system. In theory after a soft tissue release, there is more 'length' to the system, and so the 'length' needs to be stabilized via a three dimensional movement pattern that creates an eccentric load, stabilizes and concentrically shortens the tissue that was just released.

Current research, specifically by Geoffrey Bove, demonstrates that we are likely improving the ability of the interfaces of tissue to slide past each other. When layers of tissue are unable to slide past each other, a cascade of events occurs which results in the tissue cross-linking together. I believe that when this occurs, if tissue is approached with tensegrity in mind, and tension in tissue is gripped at a tangential angle, we can improve the ability of tissue glide. Self-myofascial release can be a good adjunct in these situations. I personally believe that changes experienced are a combination of both processes, depending on the context. Sometimes tissue is un-'kinked' from other tissue, while other times the relief felt being driven more from the nervous system, changing our perception and ability to connect effectively with that tissue. In cases where the same area needs to continually be released, the initial relief felt is more CNS driven rather than a 'soft tissue release'.

For example, the client with insidious lateral knee pain often will benefit from self-release to the quad/rectus femoris border, as well as the quad/ITB and to increase tissue glide. Those that experience exquisite tenderness when self-releasing these areas, particularly when the tenderness is asymmetrical from one side to the other, may benefit from this type of work for a distinct period of time. However, people often feel the need to release a specific area of the body continually, and in this case the relief obtained is from a neurological response, especially the analgesic effect documented in literature.

Fascia provides structure & tension for the sympathetic NS to either upregulate or down-regulate, as the nervous system always works toward achieving homeostasis. The sympathetic NS is responsible for flight or flight response, and requires the ability of a muscle to push and pull off its fascial surroundings, and tension is required up to a point. However, heightened sympathetic system stimulation, or suppressed parasympathetic stimulation creates prolonged tension, which potentially could affect the fluidity and ability of the connective tissue to slide past other tissue. It also could result in tighter tissue and a stronger connection to the nervous system, specifically the Motor Control Center. This connection potentially inhibits the nervous system's ability to connect to other regions, making the consideration of inhibition/facilitation and reciprocal inhibition relationships that much more relevant. If the length tension relationship of the joint is altered, over time a stress strain pattern develops where tissue on one side of the joint works harder than the tissue on the other, often times resulting in altered connections to the Motor Control Center.

Reciprocal Inhibition is generally defined as a neuromuscular reflex where muscles on one side of a joint accommodate the contraction of the muscles on the other side of the joint. This is accomplished by a decrease, or inhibition, of the neural drive to the region rather than a simple on or off switch.

For example, when the bicep flexes the elbow, the nervous system inhibits the triceps from fully firing (which would extend the elbow) in order to allow smooth and uninterrupted movement. However, sometimes these relationships become too ingrained into the system and alters otherwise normal function. This leads to the perpetuation of a negative feedback loop and dysfunctional movement patterns, and while these relationships are expected, there's a point of diminishing return. Understanding this concept, and more importantly having a strategy to address these dysfunctions, allows a more specific intervention and direction for progression.

NEGATIVE FEEDBACK LOOP PREVALENCE IN DYSFUNCTION

Mirriam Webster defines negative feedback loop in biology as "a reaction that causes a decrease in function, occurring in response to come kind of stimulus. It often causes the output of a system to be lessened, so the feedback tends to stabilize the system." Most people that are in pain are stuck in some sort of negative feedback loop, in my opinion, interchangeable with an inflammatory cycle and cumulative injury cycle.

Often I see people who have lower neck/upper trap pain and 'tightness", especially with overhead movements such as putting away dishes. These often are the people who sit at a desk doing computer work, probably at a poorly designed workstation. They demonstrate poor positioning with quiet stance, and often describe themselves as "stressed" and/or "so busy" at work. In his book *Corrective Exercise Solutions to Common Hip and Shoulder Dysfunction* Dr. Evan Osar, DC states, "When there is optimal co-activation between functional antagonists, there is maintenance of the joint position. In the presence of muscle inhibition, one or more of the functional agonists become dysfunctional and the joint is pulled in the direction of the functioning muscles. This alters the joint position as well as the instantaneous axis of rotation, thereby compromising joint stability" (p 32). What this means to me is that when there is movement dysfunction or poor positioning in posture, often times muscles on one side of the joint work harder than muscles on the other side, setting up dysfunction.

Another plausible explanation for immediate short term changes seen with tissue manipulation is the stimulation of sensory fibers including Pacinian corpuscles, ruffini endings and interstitial fibers that affect the ANS, normalizing intrafascial cell activity and normalizing the system's ability to fire without inhibitions of the track and sequence. The reality is pain alters the nervous system, and Kankaanpaa et al. (1998) and O'Sullivan (1997) have proven that low back pain can create imbalances in the activation patterns of global muscles, particularly inhibitions in the glut max and glut med, and often substituted by the biceps femoris, iliopsoas, TFL, and adductor muscles. (The vital Glutes, John Gibbons p 98). In layman's terms, this means that pain can easily inhibit muscles as a response to alterations to the nervous system. The question then becomes, so what, what to do about it?

Historically, the most successful practitioners of myofascial release respect both paradigms and are able to change the soft tissue and retrain the CNS to ensure that the changes 'stick' and are longer lasting. Robert Schleip, Ph.D., said, "this global system for rapid body regulation is inseparably connected to the endocrine and immune systems, and it also works with complex feedforward system dynamics. A "tropical wet jungle" that is a self-regulatory field as opposed to a hard wired electric cable system. Like a jungle, the brain must be continually "watered" in order to thrive or learn new movement patterns (neuroplasticity) instead of being able to plug into a cable system once and have the new information for always." For the system to integrate a new motion successfully, a movement pattern must be simple and repeated throughout the day, combining neuro and somatoplastiity, or what Lorimer Mosley, Australian Physiotherapist and pioneer in pain science (Explain Pain), calls Neuro-Bioplasticity.

Neuroplasticity can be defined as the capacity of the brain to change its structure. This is accomplished in various ways. For example the brain changes with experience and continues to do so throughout life, both positively and negatively. Think about the difficulty in learning a new task and the awkwardness involved. Some people tend to get 'worked up' when they can't complete the task with ease, while some people hardly react and are quite mindful about what they're doing. In both examples, a new task is much more difficult and awkward than one that has been done before, however, it's how they reacted to the stressor of a new activity that is habit. These are examples of neuroplasticity, and evidence demonstrates that anything we ever do reinforces, either positively or negatively, the way in which our brains function.

KEY CONCEPT: Neuroplasticity--the capacity of the brain to change its structure.

When pain persists over time, the brain begins to function differently, as the neural networks responsible for providing the experience become dysfunctional, often times becoming sensitized, meaning they require less stimulus to initiate a response. Moseley and H. Flor wrote that "the combination of sensitization and disinhibition drive systemic change in the response profile of neurons that represent the body." What this means is that the nervous system's ability to suppress incoming 'danger' signals to amplify which begins to reorganize the way in which the brain receives input from the body (Flor H, Braun C, Elbert T, Birbaumer N, Extensive reorganization of primary somatosensory cortex in chronic back patients. Neurosci Lett 1997; 224 (1) 5-8).

In other words, they don't possess the cortical mapping required to effectively perform the activity, and it needs to be remapped (or remylenated) to make changes to the motor control center. An activity that should be relatively simple but accurately reflects this is in the ability to move your toes, as the 1st toe should move separately from 2-5 and vice versa.

Clinically, I've found those with foot pain, or who have had foot pain, often times are unable to move their big toe independent from toes 2-5, and vice versa.

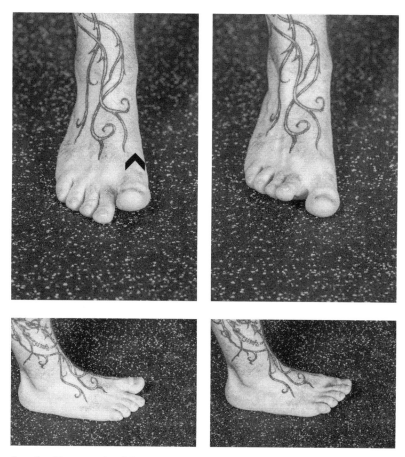

One should possess the ability to move the first toe independently from 2-5, and vice versa. If this can't be performed, there is opportunity to improve the representation of the somatosensory cortex region of the brain.

One SHOULD be able to accomplish this task without the other toes moving, and also without compensation. Those that aren't able to often times have weak intrinsic muscles of the foot, and/or don't have the body map with the brain and Motor Control Center for moving that region of the body independently. This movement can be taught, but it takes time and mindfulness to accomplish. As one is able to perform this activity, strengthening the foot muscles becomes easier, as does taking someone out of the pain pattern they might be in, and the less dysfunctional the foot becomes. If one doesn't have the independent movement in that or any region, creating the space in the motor cortex requires frequent, low intensity, and mindful repetitions in order to make neural connections. The primary goal in teaching someone a new skill is to first suppress the sympathetic nervous system, or stimulate the parasympathetic nervous system.

KEY CONCEPT: Primary Goal in teaching a new skill is stimulation of the parasympathetic nervous system.

Additional Reading

Myers, Thomas W. Anatomy Trains: Myofascial Meridians for Manual and Movement Therapists.

Lindsay, Mark, and Chad Robertson. Fascia: Clinical Applications for Health and Human Performance.

Stecco, Luigi, John V. Basmanjian, and Julie Ann Day. Fascial Manipulation for Musculoskeletal Pain.

Scarr, Graham. Biotensegrity: The Structural Basis of Life.

Osar, Evan. Corrective Exercise Solutions to Common Shoulder and Hip Dysfunction.

Weinstock, David. NeuroKinetic Therapy: An Innovative Approach to Manual Muscle Testing

Schliep, Robert. www.somatics.de

Gray, G. Functional Video Digest Series. Vol 3.6 Tweakology; Vol 4.5 The Matrix System

Bove, Geoffery, https://www.researchgate.net/profile/Geoffrey_Bove/publications

Chapter 6

Injury

Cumulative Injury Cycle, Negative Feedback Loop & Inflammatory Cycles

D r. Michael Leahy, DC, developer of the soft tissue management system Active Release Techniques, described The Cumulative Injury Cycle (CIC) as the result of dehydration, acute injury, repetitive trauma, and constant compression and tension on nerves, muscle and bones. Often the initial injury that spurs this cycle is an acute injury where there is torn myofascia. This causes immediate inflammation with white blood cells, fibrinogen secretion, and the formation of adhesions, and if not treated this process continues and the cumulative injury cycle begins. Often the CIC is the result of repetitive motions that cause more trauma and stress to tissue, which causes more inflammation and more stress, leading to a downward spiral and ultimately causing tissue to become weak and/or tense.

Cumulative Injury/Negative Feedback Loop

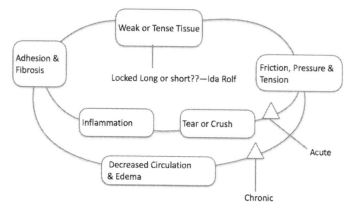

The cumulative injury cycle can also be seen as a negative feedback loop. Ida Rolf spoke about tissue being locked long or locked short. Inflammation is a normal process in the body, and often times when one is stuck in an inflammation, or negative feedback loop, the trick to breaking the loop can be to mindfully inflame the tissue more in order to continue to the stalled out process. Fluid pooling results in a cascade of events that binds the tissue to that which is around it.

For example, earlier we discussed Mary, the grandmother of 2 that was in a car accident and 2 years later still had pain. What wasn't discussed previously is that she was stuck in this CIC, which, in my opinion, can also be considered a negative feedback loop. I believe her nervous system was functioning more in a sympathetic state rather than parasympathetic, so the first objective became to 'put her fire out'. This is in order to get the body into a parasympathetic state, recognizing that lasting changes will be more likely to occur if this is the case. Her lack of posture awareness, combined with fear, avoidance of movement, and anxiety of the situation was influential in her CIC, and so her first work was to make her aware of her state of being. This was accomplished first by educating her on the process her body goes through each time she stresses out about her situation, including education about the sympathetic vs. sympathetic nervous systems. This, along with teaching her to belly breathe, was the first step to breaking the negative feedback loop Mary was stuck in. The next step was to systematically create slightly more inflammation of the tissue in order to stimulate the process of inflammation removal via tissue movement and pumping. This was accomplished via gentle soft tissue mobilization to the neck extensors and movements that engaged the neck flexors to balance out her posture. The combination of specific movements had positive effects, including creating extensibility of the tissue, allowing a differentiation of pressure within the tissue, allowing increased flow of fluids. It also helped Mary to gain confidence in pain-free movement and that she CAN make changes to her situation through mindfulness and specific movement.

KEY CONCEPT: One clinical pearl I teach my patients is that respiration is subconscious, but breathing is conscious. We respire over 20,000 times per day on average. How many of us breathe in our day? Breathing can be linked to stimulating parasympathetic response and helps to create behavior change.

A variety of factors can affect the Cumulative Injury Cycle including smoking, diabetes, and hormonal changes, as well as lifestyle factors; however, the cycle is perpetuated in predictable ways. These factors tend to increase tension in the system by creating an environment where the body is sympathetic in nature (flight or fight) instead of parasympathetic (rest and digest) and perpetuates the "weak-and-tense" factor of the cycle. The CIC has two possible routes, the inflammatory cycle and the chronic cycle, and each is independent of the other but can run concurrently.

The CIC often worsens slowly over time, typically in a manner of progression followed by a setback, worsening the injury. Over time, a downward spiral creates a chronic inflammatory environment that is self-perpetuating. Examples of cumulative injuries that lead to this cycle include carpal-tunnel syndrome and "itis's" such as epicondylitis, tenosynovitis, myofascitis, bursitis, peripheral-nerve entrapment, and thoracic-outlet syndrome. The CIC can result in a lack of inter- and intra-muscular slide, myofascial restrictions and scar tissue.

Lateral Elbow Pain Example

For example, we discussed the person with lateral elbow pain that has poor posture and also limited awareness of how he sits and moves in space that also has a numbing, possibly from nerve entrapment at the scalenes. We discussed that this patient has a tight and overactive pectoralis minor, which can lead to changes in the nerve's ability to move through tissue. This is another example of the cumulative injury cycle and also negative feedback loops at work. This person is positioned poorly, likely without realizing it, which feeds into his dysfunction. Poor sitting position combined with limited awareness of the poor positioning creates a consistent low level irritation of tissue. In addition, the tissue on the front of the body is imbalanced relative to the tissue on the back of the body because forward head and rounded shoulders increase tension into the lateral elbow. This person has low level and consistent irritation throughout chains of fascia, creating a situation where movement is aggravating, and therefore limited. However when they HAVE to move, it hurts, causing irritation and more fear of movement. Both the physical and emotional stressors creates anxiety about their situation, releasing cortisol and creating a sympathetic nervous state that continues the cycle. The approach to treatment with this type of patient has to be multifold and include working with the injured tissue and also educating about the process and cycle she is stuck in.

This patient was assigned self-release to the tissue and also stretching exercises directly for the wrist/elbow complex, in addition to posture awareness and breathing exercises. Part of the approach with this patient must be to educate them on when they don't know they're in a poor position. In this instance, we broke the CIC by soft tissue mobilization to the tissue in order to get fluid to the tissue so as to stimulate the inflammation cycle to carry the waste product found in the tissue away. We also made him more aware of his positioning by utilizing Rocktape kinesiology tape to tape the skin. Taping the skin affects the afferent input into the brain and alters the efferent output to make someone aware when they aren't in a good position. In short, the tape is applied so that when the person goes into a poor position, the tape is tensioned and the person feels the tape, making them aware of their poor positioning.

Note that we worked tissue on both sides of the joint, not only the irritated wrist extensors because the site of the injury isn't the cause of the injury. Through balancing the joint and tissue on both sides while addressing the nervous system, an environment was created to affect the mind and body. Motion and awareness of positioning will be preserved via regular specific stretching, and overall tissue stress will be decreased by posture awareness.

KEY CONCEPT:

To break an inflammation or negative feedback loop, often times the answer is to inflame the tissue further in order to facilitate the healing process while concurrently making behavioral changes. In a negative feedback loop, often times they don't know they don't know until it is brought to their awareness. Once they know they don't know, the process to integration and behavioral changes can occur.

Differentiating types of limitations: Joint pain or muscle pain or nerve pain

Clinically, it's necessary to clear a joint restriction prior to addressing soft tissue restrictions because during movement bones making up the joint need to dissociate synchronously, meaning one bone needs to move faster (or slower) than the bone next to it. If there is a capsular restriction and a bone can't move independent of the other, then the motion becomes asynchronous and a situation arises where something above or below often will have to do too much. Another way to say it is that there is interdependency between bones and joints instead of independency.

When assessing movement, addressing closing angle pinch and binding in the joint is a good first place to start. The closing angle of a joint is defined as the regressive angle, rather than the progressive angle, meaning with elbow flexion the biceps is the regressive side and the triceps is the progressive side. .

If there is capsular restriction, clearing this first is important, because joint independence needs to precede joint interdependence. I describe the joint and capsule as space between bones with plastic or shrink wrapping the bones in 360' so that they can slide, glide and roll against each other. This is the joint capsule. Restricted joints often exhibit diminished range of motion (ROM), as well as significant reduction in the ability of one bone to 'play' or move against each other. Even a joint that moves within a full ROM may exhibit premature binding, and a limitation of the ability of *tissue* to move through its full range. Active motion and also palpation can reveal areas of tissue that are grabbing, stiff and boggy as fascial strains and kinks limit the utilization of the full movement potential.

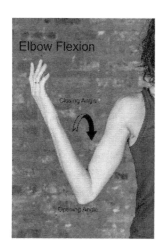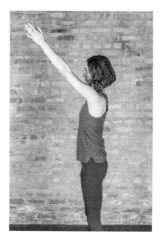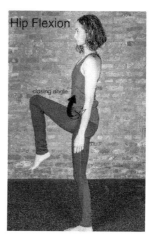

Closing, or regressive joint angle pain and pinch is often indicative of capsular limitation.

A primary objective for any movement practitioners is to create as many degrees of joint freedom as possible in order to ensure clean, pain-free and functional movement. If a joint is restricted, then the ability for a bone to synchronously dissociate is diminished, in turn creating a situation where something else overworks. Dr. Andreo Spina, DC, creator of Functional Range Conditioning says, "joints need independence before interdependence." This is a powerful statement because for there to be true freedom of movement, all joints need to move free and independent of other joints. Often joint motions become interdependent on another joint moving which leads to dysfunction.

For example, people with shoulder dysfunction (tendonitis) link, or chunk end range glenohumeral motion with spinal extension. This patient experiences binding on the top of the shoulder during shoulder flexion, indicating interdependency between the glenohumeral joint and scapulothoracic joint at end range shoulder flexion.

Clinical correlations suggest that this scenario, including a closing angle pinch, can set up an alteration of the neural drive to the tissues surrounding the dysfunctional joint. Understanding if compression or distraction changes the ability of a muscle to engage in a muscle test directs the course of treatment and 'homework for the client'. Ultimately restoring joint mobility is the first step in a movement restoration program, followed by one then two joint muscles.

SELF-ASSESSMENT: A self-assessment strategy to demonstrate appropriate glenohumeral independency is to stand with your back against the wall and flex the shoulder. The shoulder should flex approximately 170' before the spine begins to move.

If this is difficult or compensation is experienced, it's indicative of the inability to dissociate the shoulder complex from the spine. Pinching or binding on the top of the shoulder is considered a closing angle joint restriction and indicative of capsular dysfunction and should be cleared first, prior to soft tissue work.

There are instances when distraction of the joint decreases the nervous system's connection with the tissue, while other times distraction creates an increased connection. Other times, compression increases the connection with the muscle, and in other situations compression creates a decreased connection; understanding the difference is very important.

For example, Jim is a 45 year old patient with right lateral hip pain. He demonstrates decreased ROM including closing angle (anterior) hip pain on flexion, and when in 0' abduction and 90 hip flexion and internally rotates has less than 10' before compensation and medial hip impinging. When the muscles around his hip are tested in the clear, meaning not against another muscle, his glut max and glut med, among other muscles, were unable to engage. However, after a long axis distraction, those same muscles were able to meet more resistance. On the other end of the spectrum, with a quick compression of the joint, those same muscles lost the ability to resist my manual pressure. In other words, he has a compressed joint that upon compression lessened the connection with surrounding muscle and upon distraction increased the connection. Therefore, my program was geared towards first distracting and creating space in the joint, followed by teaching the nervous system to utilize the new ranges.

However, if those same hip muscles upon compression increased the connection and upon distraction decreased the connection, the exercise prescription and manual work would have been less about creating space in the hip and more of creating full range of motion. This will be progressed over time and along with ROM within a non-pinch closing angle range, and will include progressive strengthening in existing range followed by slowly increasing the joint space based on thresholds.

I believe the above situation occurs when the body craves stability, rather than mobility. The hip was tight for a reason, yet it's more of a neurological tightness versus a structural tightness. In this case, the best course of treatment would be to strengthen all the muscles that surround the joint and not distract the joint because the body is seeking stability. Conversely, if the muscles surrounding the joint came back online after distraction, then mobilizing and distracting the joint becomes the best course of treatment.

Case Study 2: Patient Presenting with Elbow Pain

In the example of lateral elbow pain, entrapment of the brachial plexus at the scalene muscles must also be considered when differentiating pain stemming from muscle, bone, nerve, or some other contributing factor. Alteration of a structure, muscle, nerve, or otherwise can change stresses and demands placed on that structure, and can be capable of affecting nerve and surrounding tissues. For example, a tight and overactive pectoralis minor can lead to changes in the way a nerve moves through tissue and can contribute, if not directly cause, lateral elbow pain. This can happen by causing other muscles in the same chain to work too hard because something else isn't doing enough. Although the site of pain is the elbow, the cause of the pain could be a tight and overworked pec minor and only by checking will we know. Performing self-myofascial release (such as foam rolling) can be of benefit for this condition. However, this alone isn't enough because the tight tissue is most likely tight due to a poorly sequenced coordination of movement in the Motor Control Center (MCC). Reprogramming how the movement is sequenced at a subconscious motor control level will accelerate the process.

Taking a step further, lack of postural awareness, combined with being good at their job creates a situation where one sits for extended periods of time, often times with a poor ergonomic work station. This poor posture and altered mechanics leads to a forward head and rounded back, an internally rotated upper extremity and an adaptive shortening of the pec minor and anterior tissue, combined with lengthening of the posterior tissue, often accompanied by extensor inhibition. Ida Rolf describes this tissue as either "locked long or locked short", and consideration of all potential sources prior to creating a treatment plan will assist one's reasoning and make a selected treatment that much more effective. In my opinion, this also fits in the paradigm of Vladimir Janda and Dynamic Neuromuscular Stabilization's (DNS) work, suggesting that upregulation of flexor muscles and inhibition of extensor muscles and must be balanced in the brain.

Fritz Perls, creator of Gestalt psychotherapy, utilized the Onion Metaphor to describe progressions of therapy, peeling away layers to get to the root of the problem. This metaphor is also appropriate to describe what it is like for people as they regain a perception of and a customization to "normal" or what has become their new normal relative to movement. Often as primary issues resolve, other issues along a myofascial chain may arise because muscles are working in new ways through larger ranges of motion. This is where importance of assessing, coaching, and recognizing the need to go slow in how and why tissue is released. Just because there is a limitation in tissue, knowing if it needs to be released right now is important information, and asking WHY is imperative. The tissue may be holding tight neuromuscularly in order to offer more stability, or perhaps is it because of kinked and adhered tissue causing the limitation. The strategies for each are different and recognizing that releasing too much too soon could result in issues the patient isn't ready for.

KEY CONCEPT: With prescription of specific movements and exercises each session, continual evaluation and updates to programs are necessary. This ensures each session is individualized based on the person in front of you that day.

Case Study 3: Midfoot Immobility to Glut Inhibition

Carrie is a 39 year old mother of 2, ages 8 and 11. She is an active runner and tennis player, strength trains 1-2 days per week, and works as an office manager of a small family owned business 25 hours a week. A few weeks prior, she began training for her third marathon and first since having children. She followed a general training plan, consisting of 2-3 'short' 3 miles runs and one progressively 'longer' weekend run. Her orthopedic history was fairly unremarkable, except for a brief period of plantar fasciitis in her left foot following both of her children, and knee pain in her left knee at random times, with no scars on her body. Recently, she presented with complaints of right hip pain that began after a particularly busy few days and weeks, when her activity and stress were more than normal.

I saw her early the fifth week of training, after 2 weeks of progressively more pain in her left lateral and posterior hip region. At that point, her complaint was a dull ache in the hip starting at 15 minutes of running that would intensify as she kept going, and would be sore for the rest of the day. She complained of a general tightness in her hip, especially after sitting, mostly along the anterior and lateral portion of the proximal thigh, which would loosen up after a few steps.

Carrie described having a fairly decent run early in the morning on Tuesday, however because of early scheduled commitments, she didn't get a chance to perform a cool down. She also drove more than normal that day because the family was going up to the cabin for a long weekend on Friday, and had to complete a few errands after work. After sleeping poorly thinking about everything she needed to get accomplish for the weekend, Carrie decided to do her second run, followed by her weekly Wednesday tennis match, which deviated from her normal schedule. The run felt normal, besides taking a little longer to feel warm, and when finished she immediately got in the car to go to tennis. Midway through the match, after lunging left for a ball and planting her left foot hard while simultaneously attempting reaching with her right hand across her body below knee height, she felt a sudden sharp pain deep in her left 'glut'. She was able to complete the match, however the pain still remained and later that night it was very achy. The next day was quite painful, and she experienced difficulty with moving around, reaching to put on her shoes, and general forward flexion, specifically in her left glut and the ischial tuberosity.

She described the initial onset of pain at a consistent 2/10, 6/10 at worst, regardless of activity. When she saw me two weeks later, the pain was a 1/10 consistently, and 5/10 at worst, however now there was pain with walking >30 minutes, or running >15 minutes. In addition, she had started getting pain with sitting extended periods, and would be uncomfortable with the first few steps after standing

Upon examination, she showed normal myotomal and dermatomal patterns, and was negative for special tests indicating lumbar pathology and facet irritation. However she did demonstrate a number of asymmetries that I believe led to the painful left gluteus complex, including an immobile thoracic spine that was right rotated, and a flatter left foot.

The following describes some specific limitations found, in the order of findings:

- Long stride:
  - ○ Limited left hip extension, demonstrated by moving around the joint rather than through the joint. When observed from posterior view, the second transformational zone of the left hip often times looks as if it's "coming back" versus the right.
  - ○ A "spin out" just after heel lift and prior to toe off on left, at second TZ.
- Squat walk: directions to client are to "walk in a room that's a little too short for you" (increases knees flex, dorsiflexion, among other things.)
  - ○ With a squat walk, she demonstrated a general rolling through the entire foot at the first Transformational Zone at heel strike, rather than a sequential dissociation rearfoot to forefoot, and also rearfoot to tibia.
- Internal & External Rotation Walk:
  - ○ Limited left hip extension, with both IR and ER walking.
  - ○ NOTE:
    - ■ When the same side hip is limited with both IR and ER gait that is a red flag for me to check to the hip capsule for limitation.
- Single Leg Squat & also Anterior Lunge:
  - ○ Limited tibial rotation noted at first Transformational Zone (TZ) versus right.
  - ○ Limited dissociation of rearfoot vs midfoot, rather there is a rolling in of the foot and knee towards middle
- Thoracic Spine Assessment: decreased overall left rotation. Also decreased right side bending, left rotation (type one motion) vs. contralateral side. This type one motion is necessary at the first TZ of the left lower extremity.
- Off weight bearing (on table)
  - ○ Closing angle pinch at 90' hip flexion, 5' adduction

- ○ Left hallux: semi-rigid
- ○ Left Midfoot: Rigid
  - ■ Cuneiforms: at rest should be positioned plantar flexed/adducted/inverted and go through the motion of dorsiflexion/abduction/eversion (the first, with a caudal translation/glide).
    - ● This motion creates the sequential dissociation in the midfoot that lengthens the proprioceptors to allow a more efficient load at the first TZ.
    - ● Unable to achieve: dorsiflexion/adduction/eversion or caudal glide vs right.
      - ○ Left foot positioned slightly flatter
      - ○ Left midfoot has tighter end feel

Muscle testing revealed a number of muscles that were weak in the clear, including the left gluteus max and gluteus medius, left posterior tibialis, left piriformis, proximal left hamstring, left iliacus, left proximal adductor, right lat and right QL. A number of these muscles work together to control the first transformational zone, and are also part many fascial lines including the Posterior X. In addition, the left glut med, left adductor and right QL are part of what NKT refers to as the Lateral Sub-System, working in synergy to stabilize the pelvis during midstance. I've often found the facilitated to inhibited relationship lies on the fascial line that works to control the movement of an intended task. The trick then becomes to identify the combinations of tissue that work to control a movement, and be able identify their relationships to each other.

Through NKT, we tied her limited midfoot mobility and compressed midtarsal joints to an inhibited glut complex, and after mobilization of the left midfoot, the glut med and max were able to fire stronger in the clear, with less pain. To be specific, the lateral glut med, along with other muscles, tested weak in the clear. When the midfoot was provided a long axis distraction and the glut med was re-tested, it tested stronger. With midfoot compression, the glut med again tested weak. When she left the first session, Carrie experienced a reduction in symptoms, and was assigned homework designed to mobilize her midfoot and synchronize her hip-foot relationship.

Specifically, her plan included mobilizing her left midfoot into the first TZ in order to gain more midfoot motion and control. Her activities, in order, were to use a towel to position her forefoot to be dorsiflexed and inverted, which is necessary at this phase of gait, followed by a left knee driver forward and to midline in order to help to dissociate the midtarsal joints. This was followed by a left leg, right 45' lunge (opposite anterior-lateral) with a left arm reach to the inside of the left knee when stepping, in order to create further dissociation at the midfoot (see picture). Last, she performed wallbangers to synchronize the foot, knee and hip while also lengthening the posterior X muscles that control the first TZ.

In the first session, I chose to focus on getting her feet moving and assign her a movement that would sync the foot with the hip, rather than focus on the hip. I went there because I was taught that if the piriformis area is tweaked out, ask "Why is the glut not controlling transverse plane motion?" That, combined with the knowledge that midfoot mobility and motion is imperative for lateral glut function, led me to working with the foot first.

When she came back 3 days later, her symptoms had increased slightly from where we last ended, but it was still better than it was prior to the first session. Her symptoms had centralized into one spot in her glut, and it was less painful sitting. Upon muscle testing in the beginning of the second visit, her glut med, left piriformis and left iliacus were the only muscles weak in the clear, which was many less versus the first session. After again distracting the midfoot, her glut med was able to fire with greater strength, and with compression of the midfoot the glut med had less ability to resist a muscle test, however neither the piriformis or iliacus muscle test changed, both testing weak in the clear.

In the second session, we began to specifically work on the left hip that impinged at >100 hip flexion, and got worse with the addition of adduction and internal rotation, mimicking the first TZ. Similar to how the midtarsal joints responded to compression and distraction, I was curious to see what happened when repeated at the left hip. With long axis distraction on the left, both the piriformis and iliacus were able to contract against greater resistance, and lessened with compression. In addition to midfoot mobility, and because her hip also responded to distraction, I chose to mobilize her left hip in supine using a mulligan strap, working to achieve the first TZ motions of flexion, adduction and internal rotation. Next, she was instructed to distract the hip utilizing a superband, followed by Functional Range Conditioning (FRC), and specifically PAILS (Progressive Angular Isometric Load) and RAILS (Regressive Angular Isometric Load) to mobilize and stabilize the new range of motion in the hips. It was performed in a seated 90/90 position (see picture). PAILS and RAILS is a patented and systematic strategy to isometrically engage muscles on the opening and closing angles of a joint in order to remodel tissue and teach the CNS to maximally, properly and safely utilize tissue in new ranges. This was followed by her midfoot mobility exercise (opposite anterior-lateral step with an arm reach), and a progression of the wallbanger to a frontal plane pivot lunge with transverse plane arm rotations (see picture). This was done to sync more dynamically and specifically the foot to the hip, and also the thoracic spine by lengthening combinations of tissue that work together during both running and tennis activities.

Her warm up prior to activity, and also at least once per day, became what we did in our session. In order that was: banded distraction of the hips utilizing a superband, then

PAILS/RAILS of hip in 90/90 position, next was her midfoot-centric exercise of left leg opposite anterior-lateral step w/ left arm reach inside of left knee towards the ground, and last was a frontal plane pivot lunge with transverse plane arm rotations. In addition, I instructed her on strategies to regress each of the motions to more easily reproduce during the day. For example, the 90/90 position can be broken out into front or back hips and performed in standing against a desk. We also educated her on the importance of frequent movement breaks during the day. This is necessary to preserve and keep new motion because motion is lotion. Also, to help become more mindful of positioning in space, and also to increase parasympathetic response in her nervous system, she was instructed to take a few deep nasal breaths (if possible), with emphasis on long, slow exhales.

There is an intimate relationship between the midfoot, consisting of the calcaneocuboid and talonavicular joints, and the lateral glut complex, consisting of fibers of the glut max, glut med, glut min and fibers of TFL. The forefoot must dissociate from the rearfoot in order to effectively lengthen the proprioceptors of the lower extremity and lengthen and tri-plane strengthen the gluts. If the foot doesn't do what it's supposed to do, when it's supposed to do it, neither will the hips or gluts. We were able to demonstrate that distraction of key joints had a positive impact versus compression, which directed a course of treatment. I believe her stiff midfoot was positioned into a relatively collapsed position, not allowing the joints to go through the act of collapsing. Bones must sequentially dissociate, particularly in the foot. This creates the required lengthening of the proprioceptors, allowing as much muscle and tissue as possible to work to control the forces presented. A bone can be in a position, such as inverted, and still go through inversion, but if the bones don't dissociate, then the joint won't feel the motion and proprioceptors won't lengthen to turn on the system effectively.

I believe that Carrie experienced her pain because of the cumulative effect of more activity in a shorter period of time. That, combined with her body running sympathetic as a response to the increased stressors in her life, resulted in a cascade of events that led to tissue trauma. Lunging for the backhand in tennis was simply the straw that broke her back, and therefore, our conversation also involved the importance of obtaining proper rest and recovering, as well as tissue tolerance and maintenance so that this injury doesn't recur.

Note: For more case studies on mid-foot, gluts, and other information, check the BioMechanical Detective channel on YouTube.

Additional Reading

Butler, D. S., & Moseley, G. L. (2003). Explain pain

Page, Phillip, Clare C. Frank, and Robert Lardner. Assessment and Treatment of Muscle Imbalance: The Janda Approach.

Rolf, Ida P., and Rosemary Feitis. Rolfing and Physical Reality

Dr. Andreo Spina, Functional Range Conditioning www.functionalanatomyseminars.com

Nickelston, P., DC. "Take the Brakes off of Movement", www.stopchasingpain.com

BioMechanical Detective Channel: YouTube

CHAPTER 7

Composition of Tissue & Scars

Collagen is very tensile and is found in fascia, bone, tendon and ligament. Elastin, just as the name sounds, has more elastic properties and is primarily found in lining of arteries, while reticulin is the least tensile and most elastic of the three and found in supporting structures around glands and lymph nodes. All soft tissue in the entire body is made up of these properties; however, it is the amount of each that changes, depending on the structure. For example, bone is made up of all four substances with the primary ingredient being ground substance with some collagen and very little of the others, while muscle has a higher concentration of elastin and collagen. Just like all cookies contain butter, sugar, eggs and flour, all tissue in the body contains ground substance, collagen, elastin and reticulin. However, what changes is the amount of each ingredient, depending on the type of cookie or part of the body.

Ground substance is a viscous gel-like material where cells and fibers lie. It acts as a mechanical barrier to foreign matter and is a medium for diffusion of nutrients and waste products. The distance maintained between adjacent collagen fibers is of critical importance to the optimal functioning and extensibility of fascia by reducing the amount of micro-adhesions that occur between collagen fibers. Often times after injury, especially when introduction of movement is delayed, the collagen fibers become crosslinked, making the sliding of various layers difficult or non-existent, and can lead to more issues. This is one reason why ensuring tissue can slide over other tissue becomes important.

Strength of connective tissue is determined by the arrangement and type of fiber and the viscosity of the extracellular matrix (ECM). The ability of tissue to slide past surrounding tissues becomes of critical importance and it's when efficient slide is hindered that limitations occur. Fibers within muscle should glide freely over one another and contract in succession (rather than simultaneously), which allows for unimpeded movement.

It is through the buffer of fascia that this gliding occurs, and if there is trauma in tissue, regardless of reason, a lack of slide may develop, leading to a cascade of events designed to facilitate protection and regeneration and create an altered relationship with the Motor Control Center (MCC). Therefore, it's important to make sure that this is addressed through our rehabilitative movements, ensuring this is addressed is imperative.

It's not enough to simply "stretch" or release a muscle or area of the body because this strategy doesn't incorporate WHY the tissue is perceived as tight. By understanding that the "tight" or painful tissue often is the area doing too much, strategies for enhancing movement can focus on areas in the kinetic chain that aren't doing enough . This in itself is different than most clinicians, who treat the area of pain in an isolated manner only. Not that that strategy is wrong, but could it be more right?

For example, rather than "releasing" the low back when painful, or stretching the low back in a manner that doesn't incorporate the rest of the system, we could give a 'Posterior X Stretch" in order to stretch both the areas above and below the low back, because the odds are the low back is moving too much because the hip or thoracic spine (or both) aren't moving enough.

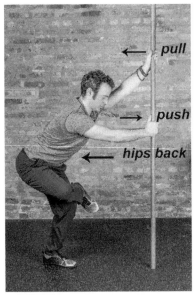

In this example, the posterior X stretch maybe assigned as a way to increase hip and thoracic motion in order to decrease low back motion. This type of stretching takes advantage of the principles of tensegrity. With this concept, the 'pushing' hand can be used to 'isolate' out a specific region of tissue within an integrated paradigm.

Scars

In the *Journal of Manipulative and Physiological Therapeutics*, Lewit and Olsanka said, "Treatment of active scars is important not only because it frequently gives excellent results but also because if active scars are left untreated, they constitute a perpetuating factor which may frustrate all our therapeutic efforts. If an active scar is diagnosed, it is essential to start treatment at the scar to assess its relevance, i.e., to decide to what an extent treatment of the scar can improve the clinical picture......."

When there is a fascial injury, there is a fascial dysfunction, and a physiological alteration in any part of the body can affect everything that is covered by the connective sheet. Symptoms can arise in the area concerned with the alteration or in an area above or below when it is not capable of adapting to the new stressor.

The reasons scars play such an important role are numerous. Bardoni and Zanier stated in 2014 in the *Journal of Multidisciplinary Healthcare*,

> "When the dermis and fascia are affected by scars, the structures are altered, and their function and capacity of interaction with the external and internal environments are lacking." The reasons are multifold and inexact, and they go on to state (p12-17) that "an excess of neuroinflammatory stimuli and a release of neuropeptides is observed, prolonging the production of growth factors, generating an extracellular matrix in excess. The neuroinflammatory overstimulation is probably a result of a reflex arc at the medullary level, which comes from the injury and then returns as a neuroinflammatory signal, with a consequent excess activity of neuropeptides. Research has confirmed an increase of nerves in the region of scarring, meaning a scar can present daily stimuli.......causing a neurogenic reflex arc."

What this means is that scarring goes way deeper than what is seen. The scar creates a response in the nervous system and lays down lots of tissue, which is an important process. However, too much of anything isn't good. The scar creates an excess stimulation and an overactive inflammatory response, creating a situation where the nervous system is sympathetic (fight or flight) and heightened.

Research has confirmed an increase of nerves in the region of scarring and an accumulation of neuropeptides. The reason for this inflammatory overstimulation isn't agreed upon, with some theories suggesting the overextension of the system, and the altered mechanical forces disrupting two types of receptors, the mechanoreceptor and the mechanosensitive nociceptor. After injury the body lays down new tissue, often times while the nervous system is heightened. The sympathetic state, combined with the haphazard alignment of the new tissue, creates crosslinking that disrupts specific nerves sensitive to tension, creating a negative feedback loop. One reason this is problematic is because the excess tension in the scars creates increased tension and alternation in the nervous system and changes the ability to connect to a muscle.

Case Study 3: Scar

One example includes a woman with a 6 year old bikini line C-section scar and has back pain, despite no "incident' to her back. Her pain typically increases when sitting for extended periods and after inactivity. Examination reveals fairly good movement overall, and she demonstrates good articulation and dissociation of her lumbar spine. However, after testing the muscles (the ability for the shortened tissue to engage in isolation) it's revealed that a number of her "core" muscles aren't able to engage properly, including the rectus abdominus, transversus abdominis, and internal obliques and multifidus on the side of pain, which is a large portion of the core. Her scar had very limited myofascial mobility, and she stated the entire scar was numb. I also observed her visible emotional discomfort w/ this area worked on, and so we began scar work simply by talking about her discomfort. She relayed how she has avoided the area because she can't feel it and it "gave her the willies" when she touched it. At that point I felt that if we jumped right into working on the scar that it would create a situation that sent her nervous system into a sympathetic state, so instead we discussed her feelings about it, and by "naming it (her anxiety) to tame it". Her "homework" began with simple breathing exercises and her laying down quietly and just rubbing her hands over her scar and pill rolling. This was in order to create a feed forward situation where she wouldn't get anxious because of the work to be done.

Once she felt a little more relaxed, we were able to verify through testing that her scar was related to the weak muscles in her core. While the exact protocol to verify the scar's relation to the muscles in her core is beyond the scope of the text (see Neurokinetic therapy), understanding that scars become upregulated in the nervous system. It's not a matter of if a scar will inhibit muscles; it's a matter of what they're inhibiting. Her homework was to release her scar in order to decrease the neural connection, followed by a subtle engagement of her Transversus abdominis in order to reprogram the firing order in her Motor Control Center.

In general, soft tissue should translate and glide freely over adjacent structures. If trauma has existed, binding down of the fascia results in abnormal pressure on nerves, muscles, bones and organs. Although still a part of the composition, scar tissue can be realigned and movement of tissue can be restored through the application of external forces such as manual therapy. If the correct process is followed, the manual therapy can also assist to reprogram the aberrant connection with the nervous system that can often cause inhibitions of surrounding tissue. Myofascial release techniques (such as foam rolling) and manual therapy can help to reestablish motion between fascial planes. It also potentially can assist to reduce fibrous adhesions and may also reestablish neural and myofascial slide and glide, while reducing the friction created by the lack of proper length tension.

An example is lateral thigh/knee pain, often called "ITB and syndrome" or snapping knee syndrome. In either case, typically the "What" of the situation is pain in the lateral thigh/knee and increased tension in the tissue. In this example, the tissue's inability to slide past itself creates a situation that 'sticks' the fascial planes together so they aren't able to slide, causing increased friction to that specific area. Self-release/foam rolling for a limited time to increase the ability to tissue to slide and glide past itself could be of benefit. However, the key is to increase a sliding surfaces ability to slide, and technique becomes important (see foam rolling guide for "pin and stretch" foam roll release).

This technique only addresses the "what" but not the "why," which always must be addressed prior to utilizing any modality. Often I see people that foam roll way beyond the point of efficacy, and so educating the clients on how repeatedly releasing is required to 'feel loose', is probably not having the intended effect. This application should only be applied for a brief period of time (weeks?) and if done repeatedly over months, the benefit to the tissue is likely minimal, and in that case there is more of an analgesic effect.

If not treated and released, the localized cobwebbing of collagen combined with the contraction of tissue results in reduced local extensibility and creates increased risk of injury along the kinetic chain.

What this means is that motion is lotion, and if you don't move it you lose it. This means that when new tissue is laid down by the body, if movement isn't introduced systematically with strategy to preserve the newly gained motion, changes to the system will be slower and the tissue isn't going to have the ability to be extensible or elastic, meaning there is a higher risk for another injury.

Prolonged immobility of tissue, typically prescribed by physicians (and often necessary after an injury) leads to situations where fresh laid adhesion creates more micro-adhesions, perpetuating the downward cascade of events. The limitation results in compensatory patterns of alternating hypo/hypermobile tissue through an entire chain, creating pain, stiffness in areas distant to the sight of primary injury, and dysfunction. A loss of lengthening potential of tissue is not so much due to the volume of collagen but to the random pattern in which it is laid down and the abnormal cross bridges that prevent normal movement.

An example is someone that is post-shoulder surgery to repair a torn labrum. This person is typically in an immobilizer for upwards of 6 weeks in order to allow the surgical tissue to heal. In this instance, initially it's important not to have the capsule stretch, however, it results in significantly reduced range of motion and an inability to move the shoulder joints independently of each other. Through compensation, it's seen that the entire complex moves as one unit.

While this is expected initially, over time each joint's ability to move independently of the other is necessary and will systematically be worked on, first through range of motion and joint mobility exercises, followed by strengthening to stabilize the motion once gotten, although they both are worked on concurrently.

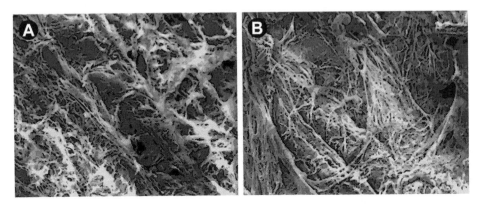

Dr. Geoffrey Bove discussed the opportunity to improve the ability of the interfaces of tissue to glide past each other, rather than "removing adhesions." This picture is an artist's rendering recreating one in an article by Dr. Teppo Jarvinen. In it, he describes how the perimysial fiber network is destroyed by immobilization, as well as the different orientations of collagen fibers. They can't be distinguished from each other in the immobilized soleus (picture B).

Characteristics of Scar Tissue

- Primarily made up of collagen
- No sweat glands or hair
- Sensitive to UV light
- Little to no blood supply
- Doesn't contain nerves
- Can't stretch or contract like regular tissue
- Approximately 20% weaker than regular tissue
- May take 2 months to a year to completely heal
- Disrupts flow of essential fluids
- More dense than regular tissue
- Creates a physiological barrier
- Trap inflammation and decrease normal channels of circulation

Additional readings

Lindsay, Mark, and Chad Robertson. Fascia: Clinical Applications for Health and Human Performance.

Scarr, Graham. Biotensegrity: The Structural Basis of Life.

Hammer, W. I. Functional soft tissue examination and treatment by manual methods: The Extremities

Stecco, Luigi, Atlas of the Muscular Fascia. www.fascialmanipulation.com

Fisher PW, Zhao Y, Rico MC, Massicotte VS, Wade CK, Litvin J, Bove GM, Popoff SN, Barbe MF. Increased CCN2, substance P and tissue fibrosis are associated with sensorimotor declines in a rat model of repetitive overuse injury. J Cell Commun Signa

Järvinen, T. A., Józsa, L., Kannus, P., Järvinen, T. L., & Järvinen, M. (2002, February). Organization and distribution of intramuscular connective tissue in normal and immobilized skeletal muscles. An immunohistochemical, polarization and scanning electron microscopic study. Journal of Muscle Research and Cell Motility, 23(3), 245-254.

Clinical Considerations

This section is designed as a guide to integrated movement options. Each body part has a brief overview of anatomy, followed by a brief description of my clinical experiences relative to each body part. In addition, there are basic movements that can be used as a jumping off point for progressions and regressions, which is based on the thresholds of the individual. While Motor Control will be discussed, specifically common dysfunctional areas, particular muscles to check for facilitations and inhibitions won't be included in the scope of this section, and I recommend you reference the book *Neurokinetic Therapy*, by David Weinstock. There is simply too much complicated information that is unique to the individual to be effectively discussed here; therefore, when appropriate, other resources will be referenced that will help to assimilate the information.

CHAPTER 8

Clinical Considerations for the Lower Extremity

Anatomy Overview

As we've discussed throughout the text, the site of pain isn't always the cause of the pain, and motion from the foot hitting the ground should be dissipated before it reaches the eyes. This means if one joint isn't able to move through its entire excursion, or range of motion, something above or below will make up the difference such as the knee or hamstring when they hurt. As physical therapist Gary Gray says, "the knee the dumbest joint in the body, and stuck between the foot and the hip", and if one of those areas isn't moving enough, then the knee is forced to make up the difference. While considering the source of the symptoms remembering the Goldilocks rule is helpful. The Goldilocks rule states that injury occurs with too much motion or not enough motion at a joint, or motion at the wrong time.

Remember the Goldilocks principle. Injury occurs when:

- There's too much motion at the joint
- Not enough motion at the joint
- Motion at the joint at the wrong time

Hip Pain: Lateral Thigh & Hip

During gait and activities including walking, running, and lunging, the lateral musculature of the stance leg during single leg stance must control the opposite side pelvis from dropping to the ground. At the first zone of gait, or what the Gray Institute calls the 1st Transformational Zone, the foot pronates, causing a reaction up the kinetic chain that requires the leg muscles to lengthen and control the body as forces are presented to it. Clinical experience demonstrates that often times, the lateral hip gets overworked because it overworks during single leg stance for too long. According to the Goldilocks principle, this situation demonstrates too much motion for too long a period of time, resulting in increased forces that are transmitted through the tissue. In other situations, the issue occurs when the hip doesn't have enough motion at the joint, and is forced to produce a lot of force without obtaining its full lengthening ability. This results in a muscle needing to produce more force without first lengthening, often causing irritation. These injuries, including IT Band pain (proximal or distal), TFL pain, glut med dysfunction and bursitis are often the victims. To assist in finding the criminals, understanding how the foot, hip and thoracic spine are moving in all three planes of motion, relative to the intended task, is imperative.

Clinically I've found those that experience lateral hip pain demonstrate an imbalance between the same side abductor and adductor musculature and contralateral Quadratus Lumborum. These three muscles work together to stabilize the pelvis in the frontal plane during single leg stance. From a motor control perspective and while muscle testing, often times one of these muscles tends to be too connected to the nervous system, creating inhibitions in the other two. Therefore balancing these relationships while creating symmetry in the ability for the hip to go through flexion, abduction, and internal rotation is a great strategy to decreasing lateral hip pain.

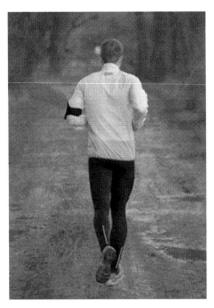

When the right leg lands, a combination of tissue, including the right quad, right glute complex, right adductors and left quadratus lumborum work to stabilize the pelvis in the frontal plane.

KEY CONCEPT:

The lateral hip is part of a number of different fascial lines that run through the body including the lateral line and posterior X line, both of which are responsible for frontal and transverse plane control respectively. Runners and endurance sport athletes alike tend to be limited in one or both of these lines. Therefore, assessing the ability to lunge successfully in the frontal plane is critical for proper function and a simple assessment can be very useful in designing a successful training and rehab program.

At what phase of gait does the hip hurt?

Check the synergy of gluteus medius, adductor and opposite quadratus lumborum.

How well does the client lunge in the frontal plane?

Does their hip go through hip flexion/adduction/internal rotation?

Movements to enhance mobility and stability of the lateral lines include:

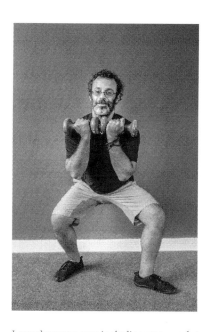 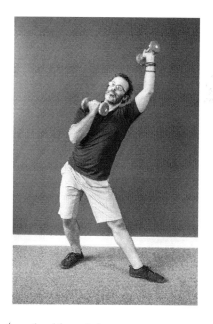

Lateral movements including staggered stance squats w/ overhead frontal plane presses are a great way to enhance the mobility and stability of the lateral lines. Presses can be multi-directional in nature.

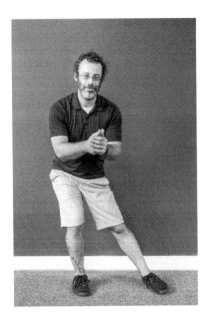

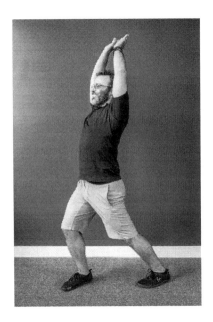

A properly executed same-side side lunge can emphasize the frontal plane component of the first transformational zone, or adduction, when performed properly. Notice that at the bottom of the motion, the hip is past the foot and knee, rather than inside the foot and knee. This allows the hip to feel flexion, adduction and internal rotation.

Common and uncommon lunges, including a frontal plane lunge with or without reaches can enhance the lateral line stability and mobility. Remember to perform motions clean, fluid and rhythmically

Case Study: The Importance of the Frontal Plane Lunge

As mentioned previously, at the first Transformational Zone (TZ), the hip should feel flexion, adduction, and internal rotation. This motion is important for maximizing gluteus complex function. Therefore, assessment is paramount, because limitation can easily lead to compensation somewhere along the kinetic chain.

One effective strategy in assessing the hips at a specific TZ is through triplane lunging. The Gray Institute describes 6 pure plane vectors in movement, specifically anterior and posterior in the sagittal plane, same side and opposite side lateral in the frontal plane, and same side and opposite side rotational in the transverse plane. Lunges can be performed in each of these planes, and a common lunge matrix is described as an anterior lunge, same-side side lunge, and same-side rotational lunge, while an uncommon lunge is defined as a posterior lunge, opposite-side side lunge, and opposite-side rotational lunge. A triplane lunge is a valuable tool for assessment. Not only can it easily mimic a Transformational Zone of a specific task, but also asymmetries can be seen when comparing one side to the other; and the addition of upper extremity arm reaches and other drivers provides more specificity.

KEY CONCEPT:

Clinically, in order to access the anterior tissue of the body, I often utilize common lunges, and to access the posterior tissue, I use uncommon lunges. However, any lunge with a specific reach can charge the emphasis of tissue load into any body part.

(A clinical note, when assigning homework to the patient, one strategy would be to have them perform movements in the plane of limitation in order to achieve more motion where they are limited. Another strategy (learned from Dr. David Tiberio, Dean of the Gray Institute) is to lunge in the plane of motion they're successful, and possibly have them reach with the upper extremity in the plane that's limited).

A lunge is simply an exaggerated step, and should be performed with synchrony, rhythm and fluidity. When movement transitions from an eccentric lengthening to a concentric shortening, it should look like a spring, rather than a shock wave. A shockwave is indicative of compensation somewhere in the system, and means there is no synchronous dissociation along the kinetic chain. Your job then, becomes to figure out where is limited. For example, the stepping foot in an anterior common lunge should feel the triplane hip motion of flexion, adduction, and internal rotation, comparable to the front foot in gait, however, the hip will feel the most flexion, compared to adduction and internal rotation because the movement is in the sagittal plane. Similarly, when a common frontal plane lunge is performed, if done correctly, the dominant triplane motion for the first TZ is adduction because the motion is lateral.

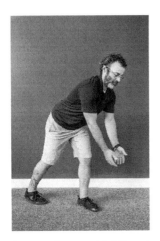 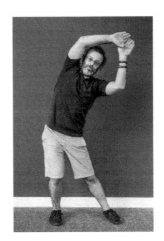 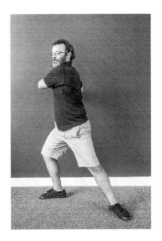

Anterior lunge with bilateral reach at knee height. A reach at the knee will emphasize more sagittal plane gluteus maximus activation, relative to a reach at shoulder height.

Same-side side lunge with opposite overhead reach. Notice the hip travels out past the stepping knee and foot.

Same-side rotational lunge with bilateral upper extremity same side rotational reach.

The reason for the inability to perform a proper frontal plane lunge will vary. Sometimes it's not in their "movement vocabulary", and once learned is easily to achieve. Other times, this motion is more difficult for people, in which case having a better idea of how the foot, especially the midfoot, and hip are working can be the key to understanding why there is difficulty. Specifically understanding if the midfoot can achieve dorsiflexion, abduction, inversion, which are the relative motions felt in the mid-tarsal joints at the first TZ. Often, the foot will be in a positioned (i.e., flat or internally rotated) and not able to go through motions that allow a sequential dissociation of the system. Dissociation, or one bone moving faster than the one above or below is necessary to lengthen proprioceptors and create an efficient eccentric load. Other times the midfoot will have too much motion, which comes with its own similar set of potential issues, and therefore understanding what is actually happening is essential. The motions can only be looked for if it's knows what should happen, therefore strategies for integrated assessment must be known in order to affect change.

Teaching a proper frontal plane lunge often difficult to learn, particularly if the movement is new. Often times, I start with a sagittal and transverse lunge, because in my opinion, they're easier to teach versus frontal plane lunges. The inability to translate the pelvis laterally outside the knee and foot at the first TZ are some of the difficulties people have when attempting this motion. Instead, the pelvis never translates outside of the knee and foot, and therefore the hip feels flexion, ABduction and external rotation (instead of flexion, ADDuction, and internal rotation). I've found that taking the time to teach the various components necessary for a frontal plane lunge, including translation and dissociation of the pelvis, and also foot placement can be beneficial and often challenging. Early in my career, I'd attempt to teach this rather innocuous, but challenging movement in the first session, however I've learned to start with success, i.e. what a client does well, rather than immediately hammer the minutia of a specific movement they aren't good at. Therefore, if one isn't initially successful with a frontal plane lunge, the frustration of attempting this and not being able to can easily lead to a sympathetic dominant response, and this should be avoided at all costs. Most times, my immediate goal is to stimulate parasympathetic nervous system response and downregulate the body, which is a reason why starting with success is so logical. A frustrating initial experience can set the wrong tone future sessions. A relatively recent realization for me is how important mindset and self-talk is in creating feedforward mechanisms in order to learn new behaviors.

Too much motion at one joint means not enough motion above or below. Another way to look at the too much, not enough scenario is: too much motion in one plane of motion can be the result of not enough motion in another plane. Understanding if a joint is too mobile or too stable is also important, and in this specific case, what plane of motion is the hip joint restricted in? I typically assess this in a number of ways, including an off weight bearing "quadrant test" to assess closing angle restrictions in the hip. My experience is that the hip will be limited into adduction, especially with a flexed hip, but it isn't consistent so don't assume! In addition, as mentioned, closing angle pinch in the hip (or any joint) is indicative of capsular restriction, and the immediate plan needs to be to focus on increasing pinch free range, which will often coincide with more ROM, less pain and more function.

If there is a compressed joint (in this case the hip), understanding how the joint responds to compression and distraction is important in directing the course of treatment. For example sometimes, upon muscle testing, distraction will allow the muscles surrounding the joint to achieve a stronger contraction, while compression would show the opposite. Other times, compression of the joint will increase the muscle's ability to contract, while distraction would show the opposite. A joint that responds to distraction will get distracted as part of the work/homework, while a hip that responds to compression will focus on joint mobility without distraction, and strengthening the muscles around the joint as much as possible. I believe that if a joint that is compressed, indicated by closing angle pinch, and responds to compression, the body is seeking stability, and doing it through compression in order to compensate for hypermobility above or below.

When teaching any movement, often times my verbal cues involve the concept of translating versus tilting. It's possible to tilt the pelvis without translating it, but it's virtually impossible to translate the pelvis without tilting. With this concept in mind, when someone has difficulty translating their hips during a stretch and instead wants to tilt, I wonder if the limitation is in the fascial chain, a restricted joint, or simply a movement that isn't in their 'vocabulary' yet. It's your job as a detective to find out. The cue "the pelvis should move further and faster than the shoulders" has been effective way to create the sequential dissociation necessary for efficient movement. Recall that if two bones move in the same speed in the same direction, the joint doesn't feel anything, and to lengthen proprioceptors and turn on the system, one bone needs to move faster or slower than another. Often times, that cue cleans up the movement, and the dissociation becomes more synchronous. Other times, the movement doesn't improve, which leads me to check for restrictions in soft tissue, joint, or both.

As mentioned, when someone has difficulty with a frontal plane lunge, I typically don't teach them how to do it in the first session or two, because it's difficult to learn. The opportunity for both the client and myself to get frustrated is high, and therefore focusing on the minutia of how to perform a small movement correctly doesn't set the right tone. Instead, I typically start with what they are good at, while also pointing out discrepancies in key regions of the body from one side to the other. Bringing awareness to something they client was previously unaware of, while also educating on the importance of creating parasympathetic responses in order to create neuroplastic changes provides a vivid illustration of why learning a new movement and *behavior* is so important. Breathing must be a part of the process. Respiration is subconscious, but breathing is conscious, and therefore taking a breath while performing this new movement allows for mind body integration, because the breath and movement are concentrated on. Breath is one pointed if focusing on the entire cycle.

When we finally do begin to introduce a frontal plane lunge, I typically utilize the following progression, which has been an effective way for someone to learn this new and rather surprisingly complicated movement. The following is a description of the regressed to progressed movement patterns that I've found most beneficial for teaching.

Standing progression to regression sequence for Frontal Plane (see Exercise Glossary for Details):

Wallbanger

Wide leg rotational squat

Wide leg small lateral step to lunge with Upper Extremity reach

Wide leg small lateral step to lunge & hold with isometric with warding pattern

Lateral lunge

Balance to lunge

Lunge to balance hope to lunge

Posterior thigh

Similar to the lateral thigh, the posterior thigh and gluteus complex in general is a crossroads of the body, involving different fascial lines including the posterior line and Posterior X. Anatomically, the gluteus complex is the thickest and most powerful muscle complex in the body. Their structure and function are interrelated, and it's apparent that the gluteus complex is the powerhouse of the body, where explosiveness is often derived from. If there is restriction in joint or tissue mobility, or if the gluteus complex isn't functioning properly, often times the smaller muscles including the hamstrings and/or deep rotators overwork and get irritated. Proper glut complex functioning is intimately involved with foot functioning and should be trained, assessed and rehabbed together whenever possible.

Movements to include when emphasizing posterior chains of the body are:

UNCOMMON LUNGE MATRIX

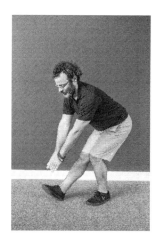 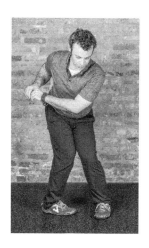 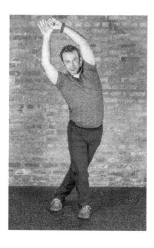

Posterior lunge, or "active hamstring stretch" which, when combined with upper extremity reaches can emphasize various parts of the posterior tissue including hamstring and gluteus complex

Opposite-side rotational lunge with bilateral upper extremity opposite-side rotational reach. Notice hips and shoulders are in-sync

Opposite-side side lunge with bilateral upper extremity opposite overhead reach.

KEY CONCEPT: Very often people present with hamstring and/or deep rotator pain of some sort, which forces the question WHY is it overworking? Why isn't the glut complex controlling frontal plane motion, causing the hamstring to overwork in some way? Why isn't the glut complex controlling transverse plane motion, causing the deep 6 (or some combination of) to control the motion? Often times the reason lies somewhere else along the kinetic chain and why understanding triplane motion for an intended task is so important. Remember to find out what the thoracic spine and foot are doing, along with the hip relative to the intended task. There is likely also tissue along the kinetic chain that can be enhanced such as the mid back and calves, which will often also be shorter than ideal and can contribute to increased hip, knee or low back motion. Increased thoracic kyphosis, which lengthens the posterior chain, could be causing posterior thigh pain just as easily as a locked up mid-tarsal joint also can.

What is the midfoot doing? How does the hip load?

A posterior lunge, and UNCOMMON lunges in general are an effective way to target the posterior musculature, particular opposite side lateral lunge. A recent study discusses the best way to load the posterior lateral glut complex is via an opposite lateral step up exercise.

When someone can't perform a lunge appropriately, a regression is a weight shift, which mimics a lunge in a more stable environment. One difference to note, is that with a weight shift, the front leg will experience a top down motion, rather than a bottom up motion.

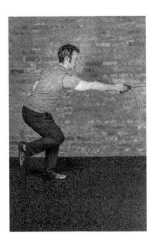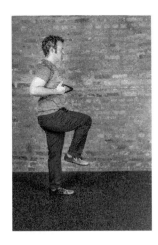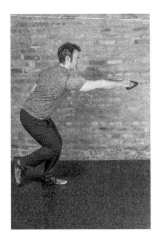

The posterior X squat<>row is a great movement to lengthen and strengthen together. This movement can be regressed or progressed by making either squat or pull end a single leg stance or toe touch support.

Medial Thigh

The medial thighs contain a group of synergists that possesses the ability to control, or limit, all sorts of motions. The adductors are the worst named muscle group in the body because in upright function they do everything except adduct the hip, as this motion is given for free when the foot hits the ground. The body needs to control the forces presented to it, and therefore depending on where the adductor group is relative to the body and axis of the hip, the medial thigh group can assist in hip extension, hip flexion, pelvic internal and external rotation, and can even control OPPOSITE hip adduction. The medial thigh region can wreak havoc to the rest of the system, contributing to pathologies including femoral-acetabular impingement, back pain, hip pain, hamstring and also anterior thigh pain.

Personally, I've discovered that those with hip capsule pathology often times demonstrate right and upregulated adductors in an effort to protect and provide stability to the system. This contributes to a situation where the femoral head glides anteriorly in the joint more than spinning, leading to other arthrokinematic issues at the joint level. Those with a femoral-acetabular impingement, demonstrating closing angle hip joint pain with hip flexion, also typically have very short and neurologically tight adductors to protect. In addition to releasing the adductors, ensuring that the hip joint has adequate roll of the head of the bone is important because this hip will lose the roll and have an increase in the sliding of the femoral head. In addition, the adductors can become facilitated or inhibited, and often times demonstrates a strong relationship to the ipsilateral abductor and contralateral quadratus lumborum, all of which work synergistically to stabilize the pelvis during single leg stance.

KEY CONCEPT: The medial thigh, or adductor group, are part of the crossroads of the body and one of the areas that are included in a number of fascial lines including the anterior flexibility highway and Anterior X.. Assessing this region for tissue length and ability to dissociate through movement is extremely relevant. Don't be afraid to put your hands on the medial thigh tissue and take the extremity through motions that affect this tissue in order to FEEL what is happening. Particularly useful are lateral and transverse plane lunges, which require a synergistic dissociation of the muscles to control the motions. Is there a symmetrical tension created under your hands during a specific motion? What does it feel like versus the other side, or does the tension develop abruptly and in one specific area?

Is there closing angle hip pain? This must be addressed prior to a soft tissue release.

Movements and Exercises to include for increase length and strength:

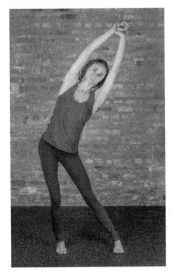

Frontal plane lunge with bilateral hand reach opposite overhead to emphasize load & length of trail leg adductors, amongst other regions.

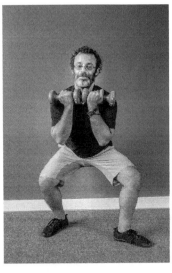

Staggered leg stance squat to press with dumbbells start.

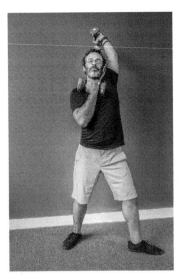

Staggered stance squat to press with alternating posterior overhead press and return.

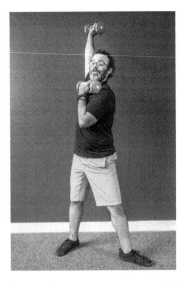

Staggered stance squat to press with alternating same-side rotational press end.

Anterior Thigh

The anterior thigh is one of those areas that tends to be chronically tight in most of western society due to our sedentary and seated posture. It also is part of the Anterior Flexibility Highway and Anterior X, and maintaining the extensibility of the anterior thigh and hip through soft tissue and movement modalities is essential for pain free living. I can think of nobody that has too much length in this part of their system, and therefore maintain the tissue extensibility in this region is important.

KEY CONCEPT:

The anterior thigh, or "front butt," as Physical Therapist Gary Gray refers to it, is part of the many fascial lines of the body. Mobility and tissue extensibility in this region is essential to maintaining good posture and vitality. Make sure to check the calf length on the ipsilateral leg, because active length of the anterior thigh, or hip extension, goes directly with ankle dorsiflexion, as to achieve full hip extension one must achieve full dorsiflexion. If one has a tight calf complex then they won't be able to fully dorsiflex, which means they will achieve heel up early in the gait cycle, leading to a hip won't ever be able to get fully extended due to the ankle never achieving full dorsiflexion. When the heel comes up at the second phase of gait, the knee flexes and causes hip flexion too in preparation of heel strike. .

Ensure hip/calf length. Is anterior hip pain felt at first or second phase of gait?

Movements and exercises to consider to enhance Anterior Thigh tissue:

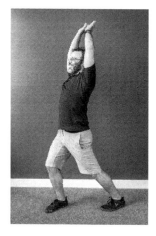

Anterior lunge with bilateral overhead reach

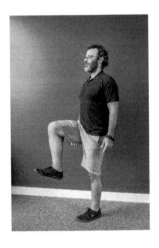

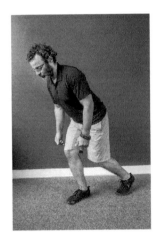

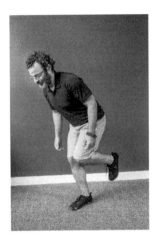

Single leg stance & balance to lunge start.

Anterior balance to lunge end, regressed (trail leg remains on ground)

Anterior balance to lunge end, progressed (trail leg foot lifted)

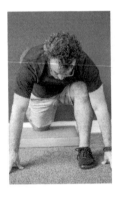

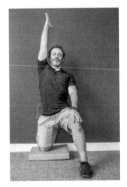

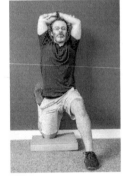

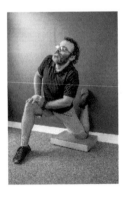

Kneeling anterior flexibility highway stretch start.

Kneeling anterior flexibility highway lunge with overhead reach.

Kneeling anterior flexibility highway stretch, progression. Notice hands overhead and head, shoulders, and hips aligned vertically.

Kneeling anterior flexibility highway stretch with compensation. Notice the unaligned head, shoulder and hips.

Knee Pain

The knee is an area of the body, similar to the low back, which takes the hit for what doesn't happen correctly at joints above or below. It's made up of primarily two major bones, the femur and tibia, in addition to the patella, which follows in the direction of the other two bones. If the hip (or foot) doesn't do what it needs to do when it needs to do it, then often the knee will be forced to make up the difference. As physical therapist and founder of the Gray Institute, Gary Gray says the knee is the dumbest joint in the body, stuck between the foot and hip with nowhere to go or hide", so a good strategy is to ensure proper triplane foot and hip motion.

Anterior-Medial Knee

Like most injuries that aren't a crush injury, anterior and medial knee often takes the hit when there is an issue at either the foot or hip. 'Patellar issues' in the anterior knee are a common source of irritation for those with knee pain, and often times stem from an asynchrony between the tibia and femur. Understanding that the patella is simply along for the ride and in most instances a victim, allows the criminal to be identified easier, and is helpful in ascertaining where knee pain is stemming from. An example of this asynchrony is illustrated in someone with a very rigid rearfoot, floppy forefoot, or foot structure issue in general. If one demonstrates a rigid rearfoot that is stuck in an inverted position often times won't be able to get the calcaneus everted as much as the contralateral side, resulting in less of a pronated end range position versus the other. The decreased pronation results in less tibial inward rotation versus the other side and therefore a biomechanical dilemma occurs at the knee, and the femur ends up rotating inward faster than the tibia, resulting in the knee feeling an external rotation moment when it should feel an internal rotation moment. Often medial knee pain, or pes anserine bursitis, occurs distal to the joint line, as the pes anserine (or goose's foot in Latin) is the intersection of the Gracilis, Sartorius and Semimembranosus; and becomes overworked when there is too much movement occurring at the tibia or femur to control rotation.

KEY CONCEPT: When someone presents in the clinic with complaints of anterior or medial knee pain evaluating the foot and hip is essential. There are 22 muscles that attach to the femur and one that attaches to the patella, in cases like patellofemoral pain and medial knee pain, think about why the knee hurts. More times than not it isn't the patella's fault that the knee is hurting, rather the patella gets smacked into the lateral side of the femoral condyle due to an external rotation moment at the knee when it should be internally rotating. This could be secondary to a foot that's not doing what it needs to do, or just as easily from a hip that is limited and so comparing both is important.

Posterior and Lateral Knee

The posterior knee has several tissues that cross the joint, as some fibers extend up above the knee and others fibers extend down below. Limitation in tissue extensibility on the posterior chain muscles can often contributes to knee dysfunction. In addition the neurovascular bundle is found in the posterior aspect of the knee, and care should be taken when palpating and working in this area of the body; and while working in this region, a good rule is move away if a pulse is felt.

In addition, the popliteus is often a muscle that becomes problematic in those with knee (or lower extremity) dysfunction, particularly after surgery. Based on the attachment points at the posterior lateral femoral epicondyle and the posterior surface of the proximal medial tibia, the popliteus is the only muscle in the lower extremity that creates the triplane motion of knee flexion, abduction and internal rotation. Another way to say it is, in isolation, this small and powerful muscle creates the tri-plane knee motion otherwise given for free when the foot hits the ground. All muscles in the lower extremity control knee flexion, abduction and internal rotation at the first phase of gait, except the popliteus. The exact reason is unclear, however I believe it's to re-sync an otherwise asynchronous movement. For example if the knee, which should feel internal rotation from the time the foot hits the ground up to and until heel rise, feels external rotation when it shouldn't, the popliteus can concentrically contract to speed up whichever bone isn't moving at the proper speed. The knee feels internal rotation at the first phase of gait because when the foot pronates (secondary to reacting to heel strike) the tibia internally rotates following the talus. This creates femoral internal rotation, but at a slower rate than the tibia because it's further from the ground, which is driving the reaction. Over time, if the femur ends up rotating inward at a faster rate than the tibia, the knee would experience a biomechanical dilemma (feeling external rotation when it should feel internal rotation), and so the popliteus can contract to speed up the tibia, potentially becoming too connected to the nervous system (or not connected enough), and causing issues up and down the myo-kinetic chain related to the particular dysfunctional movement pattern.

KEY CONCEPT: Clinically it is often seen that the posterior and lateral knee get angry and dysfunctional when there is a limitation in the foot, hip or thoracic spine. Ensuring proper length of the posterior and chains is essential to maintaining healthy knees. Remember that the knee is stuck in the middle with nowhere to go. The knee is the foot/ankle because they are both made up of the tibia, just as the knee is the hip because they too are made up of the femur. In addition, in runners the posterior chain often is an issue, because as people run longer distances they succumb to gravity and begin to lean forward. When this happens, the thoracic spine increases the kyphosis, the hips and knees will respond by flexing, which puts more forces through the knees.

-Related to the posterior flexibility highway & Posterior X
-Check knee internal rotation at the first and second phase of gait (prior to toe off)
-Check the thoracic spine mobility. People with posterior knee pain, especially runners, walkers and bikers, lack thoracic mobility overall, particularly into segmental thoracic extension.

Movement and exercise considerations for posterior knee include:

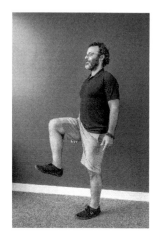

Balance to lunge start & end

Note, during stance phase, this movement emphasizes the posterior line and stance leg. During a lunge, to emphasize the posterior knee, keep the stance leg heel on the ground.

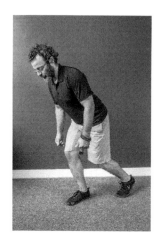

Anterior balance to lunge, regressed.

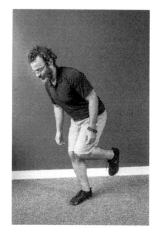

Anterior balance to lunge, progressed.

The balance phase emphasizes the posterior stance leg, in addition to other muscles.

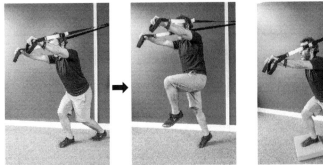

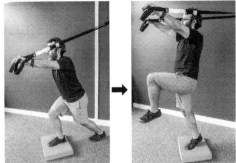

Suspension strap intrinsic foot, start, end

This motion emphasizes core stability and active eccentric loading of the posterior stance leg musculature.

Suspension strap single leg eccentric start and end, progressed with blue airex pad.

Anatomy Overview

When looking at the muscles that attach at the calf and ankle, I think of "local road" muscles, or intrinsic muscles that cross one or zero joints, and "interstate highway muscles", crossing one or more joints in each of the three compartments that make up the calf. The anterior compartment includes the anterior tibialis, extensor hallucis longus, extensor digitorum longus and peroneus tertius, while muscles in the lateral compartment are comprised of the peroneus longus and peroneus brevis. Muscles in the posterior compartment of the leg are divided into the deep and superficial muscles. The superficial muscles include the gastrocnemius, soleus and plantaris, while the deep muscles include the flexor digitorum longus, the flexor hallucis longus, the posterior tibialis and popliteus. To me, the calf is a complex, working together along with the 26 bones, 33 joints and 34 muscles of each foot to control the body in space. Thinking in terms of which phase of gait is more limited is helpful to identifying which fascial line wan be worked and enhanced.

Outside Ankle

The muscles on the outside of the ankle include the peroneus (or fibularis) longus and brevis. In isolation the muscles plantar flex and evert the ankle and calcaneus and in integration work eccentrically to control the first ray at the back phase of gait while it has to stay anchored to the ground. These muscles are fascially connected into the lateral highway, as well as into the Posterior X by way of the fibular head attachments of the biceps femoris.

KEY CONCEPT: If pain is located in the outside ankle, be sure to check the lateral and posterior X highways for dysfunction, as often limitation or pain in the outside compartment of the ankle is correlated with dysfunction up the kinetic chain, particularly amongst these highways. Clinically, transverse & frontal plane pivots are a powerful movement/exercise that can add a lot of mobility & stability to this and other regions.

Inside Ankle

The inside of the ankle houses a lot of tissue that travels from the back of the tibia, deep to the superficial calf muscles including the gastrocnemius and soleus. From the back of the tibia, the tissue runs down the inside of the shin and into the bottom of the foot. Often times, this area, including the posterior tibialias and deep toe flexors, become stressed out from too much load to the tissue for too long a period of time, often pronating too long during the gait cycle. Be sure to check the midfoot for the ability to unlock at the first phase of gait, and lock at the second phase, because issues at either zone will greatly affect these muscles.

KEY CONCEPT: Clinical experience dictates that often times the bottom of the foot begins to hurt when there is too much load into the tissue. The question becomes, WHY is there too much load? It's important to remember that when the foot hits the ground it needs to be a mobile adaptor and when it is the rearfoot about to toe off the foot must become a rigid lever. If the midtarsal joint isn't able to lock up in the appropriate manner then the body is forced to propel off an unstable and unlocked midtarsal joint and pain arises. The key is to recognize that the midtarsal joint has difficulty locking and if that is the case it is recommended to that referral to a healthcare provider for further testing could be recommended.

Foot Pain: Anatomy Overview

The foot isn't just one big bone, in fact between both feet, ¼ of all the bones in the entire body are found there. Each foot has 26 bones, 34 muscles and 33 joints that together allow the foot to be a mobile adapter when it is striking and collapsing into the ground and a rigid lever when the foot is the rear leg in order to provide a stable surface for the muscles of the foot and leg to propel forward. Typically in order to simplify the analysis of the foot, it is analyzed as the first ray/big toe, the forefoot and rearfoot division, called the midtarsal joints, and the rearfoot, called the subtalar joint. Together these parts of the foot work to ensure that the foot is mobile and stable enough to perform all of its functions. Ensuring each section of the foot is able to work at the 2 zones of transformation related to gait is important. In addition tight tissue here, or up the posterior aspect of the calf can greatly affect hip functioning, so these two areas should be trained and treated together whenever possible.

KEY CONCEPT: Anyone that has bottom of the foot pain is also going to have dysfunction in the medial compartment of the shin. It's important to understand that this tissue is responsible for eccentric load of the foot during pronation and too much or not enough motion causes stresses not only to the tissue on the inside but also the bottom of the foot and even up to the hip.

KEY CONCEPT: "When the foot hits the ground, everything changes" is a common saying in the rehabilitation worlds, and accurately describes the thought of how important the foot is to optimal function, affecting local parts of the body as well as regions of the body far away from the foot such as the opposite shoulder. All Flexibility Highways start in the foot and understanding the basic function of the foot is critical to pain free activity. Because the foot is such a challenge and intricate area of the body, if one experiences continued pain in this region it is recommended to see professional advice in order to properly treat the dysfunctional and/or painful area.

Movement and exercises to lock mid-tarsal joint in preparation for toe-off:

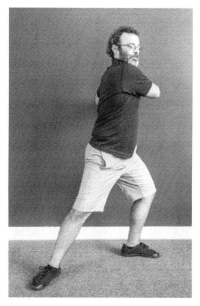 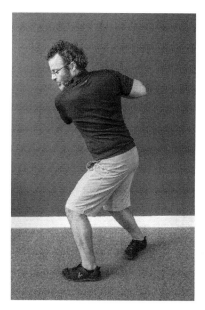

Rotational pivot squats are good for eccentric load of the anterior and posterior chains of the body, in addition to being beneficial for balance, strength, and getting the mid-foot to go through loaded motion.

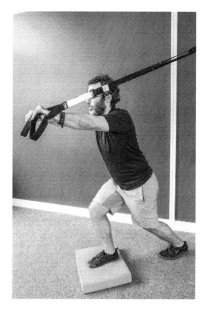 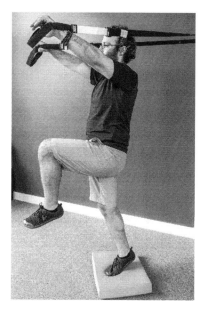

Suspension strap single leg toe off with blue airex pad, start and end.

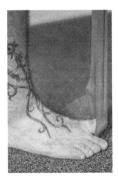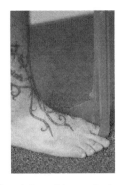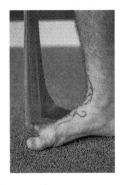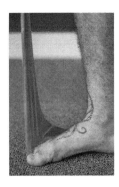

Isolated toe flexor strength training with exercise band start, end

Those with weak intrinsic muscles often demonstrate difficulty moving the big toe separately from 2-5, and vice versa. When this is the case, in addition to strengthening the intrinsic toe muscles, creating space in the brain is important in order to better connect with the region. Progressions for intrinsic foot muscle strength include suspension strap squats.

Movement and exercise considerations: Sagittal, Frontal & Transverse plane pivots

Frontal plane pivots, starting with a same side, side-lunge and ending in an opposite side, side-lunge is an effective way to target the outside of ankle musculature; in addition to utilizing a transverse plane pivot.

TRANSVERSE PLANE PIVOT

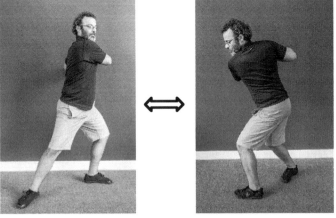

Rotational pivot squats are good for eccentric load of the anterior and posterior chains of the body, in addition to being beneficial for balance and strength.

Same-side lunge & opposite-side lunge, when taken from one into the other is called a pivot. In this combination, triplane pivots are performed with hands into or away from the stepping leg. Pivots are useful to strengthen and lengthen a chain in integration, while also working balance and "core" strength because moving the legs and arms forces the middle to react and control the motion.

FRONTAL PLANE PIVOT

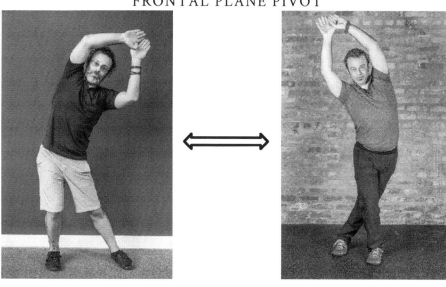

Same-side side lunge with bilateral hands opposite overhead reach

Opposite-side side lunge with bilateral hands opposite overhead reach

OR

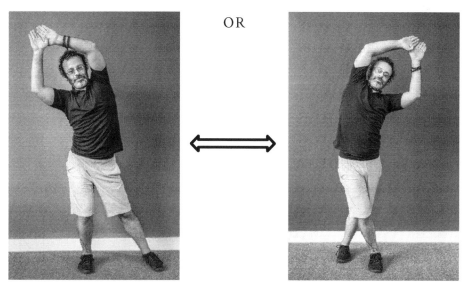

Same-side side lunge with bilateral hands same-side overhead

Opposite-side side lunge with bilateral hands same-side overhead

SAGITTAL PLANE PIVOT

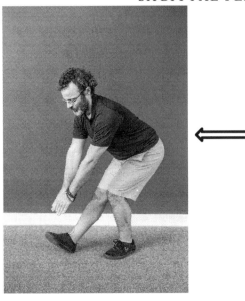

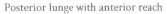

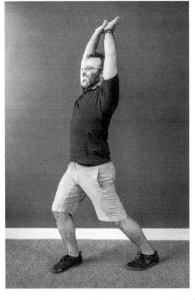

Posterior lunge with anterior reach

Anterior lunge with posterior overhead reach

UNCOMMON LUNGE VARIATIONS

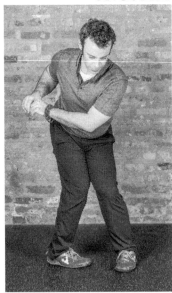

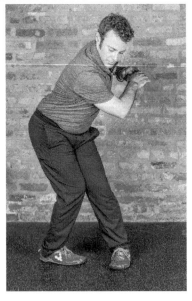

Opposite side rotational lunge with bilateral upper extremity opposite side rotational reach. This movement creates motion where the hips and shoulders are in-sync.

Opposite side rotational lunge with bilateral upper extremity same side rotational reach. This movement creates motion where the shoulders and hips are out-of-sync.

Movement and exercise considerations for this part of the ankle

Triplane pivot activities (see above)

Self-Myofascial Release Work

Physiological effects of self-myofascial release

- enigma of good hurt
    - Soft tissue work can be very uncomfortable, bordering on the point of becoming overwhelmingly painful and at the same time also "hurt so good".
    - Concepts of overdoing it
        - Two types of patients
            - Please do what I ask you to do
            - Please don't' overdo it because you'll cause more damage

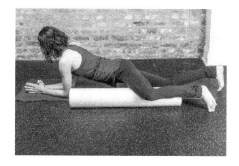

SMR medial thigh, start

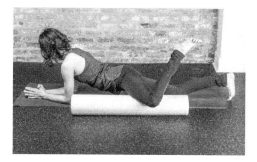

SMR medial thigh, end

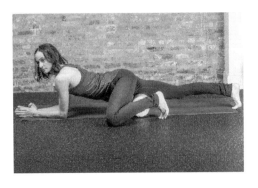 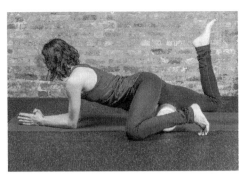

SMR anterior thigh, start   SMR anterior thigh, end

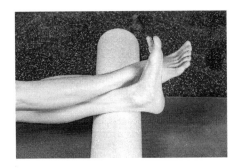 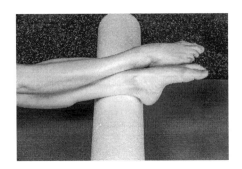

SMR calf, start   SMR calf, end

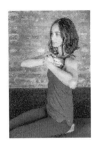 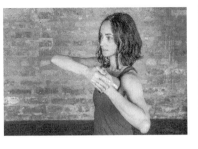 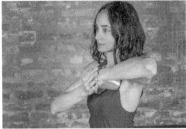

SMR anterior chest, start   SMR anterior chest, end

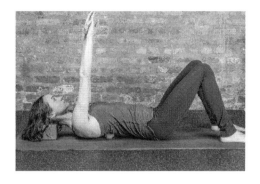
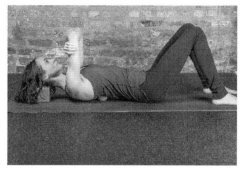

Thoracic spine, start   Thoracic spine, end

Note: With thoracic spine SMR, two tennis balls are taped together into a "peanut" shape and one ball is placed on each side of the spine.

Additional Reading List

Root, M. L., Orien, W. P., & Weed, J. H. Normal and abnormal function of the foot.

Osar, Evan. Corrective Exercise Solutions to Common Shoulder and Hip Dysfunction

Gray, G. Functional Video Digest Series. Vol. 1.1 The Knee. Vol. 1.5 The Hip: 3D Power Vol 3.4 Functional Manual Reaction- The Foot and Ankle, Vol. 3.8, www.GrayInstitute.com

Iyengar, B. K. Light on yoga: Yoga dipika

Desikachar, T. K. The heart of yoga: Developing a personal practice. Rochester, VT: Inner Traditions International.

Wolf, Chuck. DVD. "Anatomy of a Lunge," www.HumanMotionAssociates.com

CHAPTER 9

Clinical Considerations for the Thoracic Spine & Upper Extremity

---

Anatomy Overview

Due to positioning, the thoracic spine (mid-back) is an area that tends to demonstrate an opportunity for improvement in just about everyone, and is amplified though our overall sedentary lifestyles. Our tight mid-backs, combined with a limited awareness of positioning in space (or proprioception), results in common areas of pain and dysfunction in the body. Poor posture is really our bodies search for comfort against gravity, possibly as a result of physical or psychological injury, or possibly because of weakness and lack of awareness of positioning.

Often times, people describe 'tightness' around the mid-thoracic/scapular area. Yet, this tissue typically isn't short and tight, rather it's long and taught. However, because of altered length tension relationships, there is the perception of 'tightness'; but most times, short tight muscles are happy that way, and rarely complain about being so. It's the long taught muscles, which are under a consistent tension, that provide the neurological perception of being tight.

Examples can be found all over the body, including around T7, where the tissue often becomes lengthened and "locked long"; a term used by Ida Rolf to describe tissue being adhered in a lengthened position to that which is around it. Other areas include anywhere that has consistently felt tight and been stretched for extended periods, with no real change, including the hamstrings and piriformis. Most times, simply stretching these regions may provide limited relief because of an analgesic response, however stretching long and taught tissues only feeds into the dysfunction. Typically change occurs through a combination of releasing the "locked long" and "locked tissue", followed by stretching the short tissue (in this example at least the anterior chest tissue) and strengthening the long tissue, in this case the parascapular muscles; combined with re-educating on proper positioning and posture.

In addition, ensuring proper movement patterning that allows proper scapulothoracic mobility is a key to relieving and preventing scapulothoracic dysfunction. I find the Anterior and Posterior X's work well to accomplish this task. Often times, people aren't aware of their positioning, and therefore behavior change and becoming aware are necessary to create lasting change.

KEY CONCEPT: Ensuring thoracic mobility, particularly into same side, side-bending and rotation, referred to as type two thoracic motion, is a powerful strategy to increase overall thoracic mobility.

Type 2 motions in the thoracic spine enhance extension. Type two motion is defined as side bend and rotation in the same direction, or together.

Thoracic-centric exercises that create the proper side bending and rotation are important. Yoga exercises including down dog and a modified "child's" pose are helpful for enhancing thoracic extension, which tends to be limited on many people due to continually fighting gravity particularly while sitting.

Down dog, modified child's pose and suspension strap lunges w/ Overhead reaches are all good ways to enhance thoracic extension

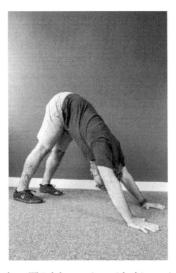

Down dog. Think long spine with this motion.

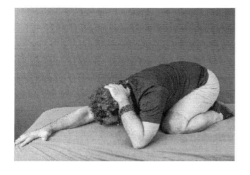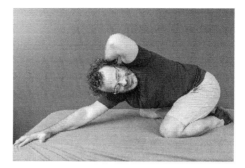

Childs pose with type two thoracic spine motion.

This modified child's pose position is good for 'isolating' the mid back. Often people with thoracic dysfunction have difficulty fully engaging the diaphragm. This movement sequence can aid in breathing more efficiently while also creating thoracic extension.

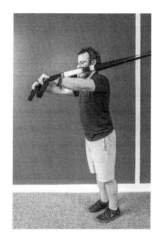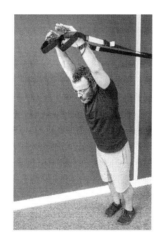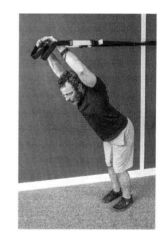

Suspension strap 'fallout' for thoracic extension, start

Suspension strap 'fallout' for thoracic extension, end

Suspension strap 'fallout' with lumbar extension compensation

Important exercises to consider, especially for those that work at a desk, includes proper ergonomic orientation, as well as movements that are geared towards enhancing the areas of the body that tend to become limited in mobility due to battling gravity, including the thoracic spine and hips.

Exercises to consider while seated at a desk include:

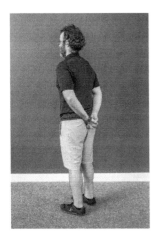

Chest Expansion, start

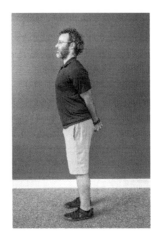

Chest Expansion, end

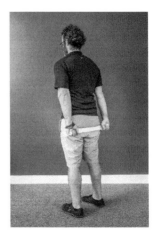

Chest Expansion, start
(alternative)

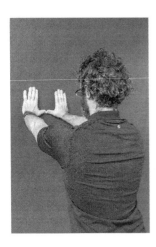

Thoracic extension against
wall, start

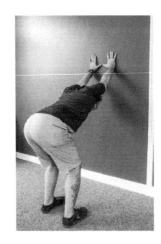

Thoracic extension with long
spine, end.

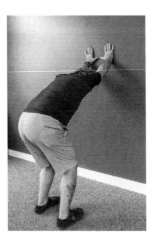

Thoracic extension
compensation.
Compensations include
increased mid-back "rounding"
or kyphosis, and or flexing
neck do head, ribs and pelvis
are not aligned.

Shoulder Pain: Anatomy Overview

Understanding that the 'shoulder' is made of four joints, the Acromio-clavicular (AC), Sternoclavicular (SC), Glenohumeral (GH), and scapulothoracic, which together form the shoulder complex is important. The scapulothoracic joint, while not technically a joint because it is the intersection of the thoracic spine and scapula, is considered a functional joint because of how the scapula slides and glides on the ribcage. There are 19 muscles attaching to the shoulder blade, and they're a combination of single and multi-joint muscles that work together and control the shoulder complex as it moves through space. The single joint muscles (including the rotator cuff) responsibility is to center the head of the humerus in the glenoid cavity of the scapula, while the multi-joint muscles regulate the extremity moving in space.

KEY CONCEPT: There are one joint muscles, analogous to local road muscles, and multi-joint muscles, which can be compared to interstate highway muscles. Local road muscles are responsible for maintaining the relationship between the heads of the bones that make up the joint, while the interstate highway muscles are responsible for moving the limb in space. Problems often occur when the interstate highway muscles do the job of the local road muscles.

Recall that musculoskeletal pain often occurs at the place that experiences too much motion, making it the victim, or area that is injured. The criminal, typically found one joint above or below, is the criminal and area where motion needs to be increased in order to improve the synchronous dissociation that all joints should feel. Creating more motion at the criminal will lessen the stress to the victim. It's also important to note that current pain science describes that often pain persists at the site of an injury long past when the tissue is healed. Typically this happens with more chronic injuries, and so educating clients on how to deal with pain is necessary because often pain cycles become prohibitive and self-perpetuating. The book *Explain Pain,* by David Butler and Lorimer Moseley is a fantastic resource to explain the pain processes that we all experience.

Anterior Shoulder Pain

Often times people with anterior shoulder pain experience some type of impingement syndrome where anterior attaching tissue rubs against a bone and gets inflamed and angry as a result of altered mechanics. This is the person with poor posture awareness that sits a lot, increasing thoracic kyphosis, protruding the head, and internally rotating the upper extremities, while shortening the hip flexors; ultimately altering the length tension relationship of the musculoskeletal system.

Clinically I've found that many times those with anterior shoulder pain demonstrate an anteriorly placed humeral head in the glenoid fossa, compared to the contralateral side. Recall that motion and position are different, and during GH flexion and abduction moments, the head of the humerus needs to translate/slide anteriorly in the joint. If positioned anteriorly, the humerus won't be able to move anteriorly with motion, resulting in impingement. Closing angle pinching with any motion and is indicative of joint restrictions, and before moving to advanced exercise/movement, closing angle pinch must be cleared. Joints need to be independent through movement rather than interdependent, and in this scenario the humerus and scapula are interdependent and coupled with movement. Moving through this pinch will only irritate tissue, and until pinching is cleared, movement progressions should be within a pinch free zone, focusing on restoring joint mobility before muscle extensibility.

KEY CONCEPT:

Anterior shoulder is fascially linked to the Anterior X fascial highway, through the same side biceps, external oblique, contralateral internal oblique, hip flexor, adductor, & posterior tibialis to lengthen and control forces in rotation and is also linked to anterior flexibility highway.

Check same side hip internal rotation, especially for throwers because if the hip is limited into internal rotation, the same side anterior shoulder often gets overloaded at the end of the loading phase in order to make up the difference of the inability to load the same side internal rotation.

Anterior shoulder pain? Check humeral head positioning

For those that have anterior shoulder pain, be sure to check the same side hip into extension, because often people will impinge in the anterior aspect of the shoulder as a compensation if they are unable to extend their hips and thoracic spine.

Ensure that each movement has a synchronous dissociation of body parts. If within the scope of practice, place your hands on specific segments to ensure there is dissociative movement.

Each movement should be clean, fluid and rhythmical.

Integrated Exercises Options for Shoulder

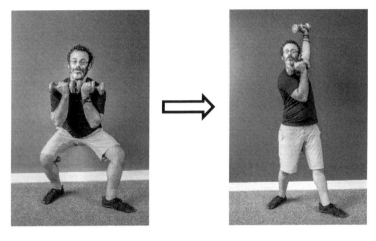

Staggered stance squat to press start

Staggered stance squat to same-side rotational press

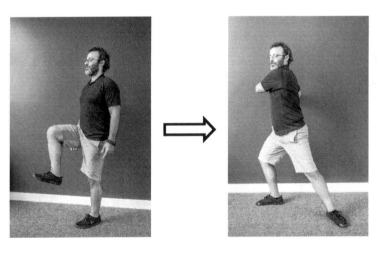

Single leg balance OR balance to lunge start

Balance to same-side rotational lunge with upper extremity same-side rotational reach end

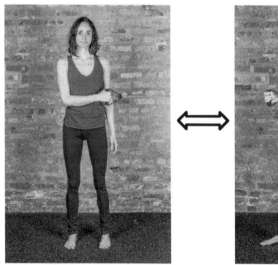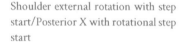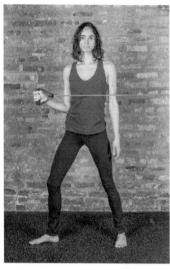

Shoulder external rotation with step start/Posterior X with rotational step start

Shoulder external rotation with same-side rotational step/Posterior X rotational step end

---

Posterior Shoulder Pain

Consistent with most soft tissue irritation, posterior shoulder pain often is the result of an asymmetrical distribution of forces through the kinetic chain and focalizes into one particular spot; in this case, the posterior shoulder. Recall, typically the site of pain isn't the cause of pain, therefore differentiating if pain is driven from irritated tissue or referred from another region of the body is important. Pain often arises in the posterior shoulder with glenohumeral abduction and external rotation, such as the cock up phase for a thrower, or when someone reaches across their body, such as a line worker that packs boxes. Therefore, determining when, how, and especially WHY the shoulder hurts for a specific task allows for a more individualized program.

Closing angle joint pain experienced with abduction and external rotation is indicative of a capsular restriction, and must be cleared prior to addressing the soft tissue mobility surrounding the joint.

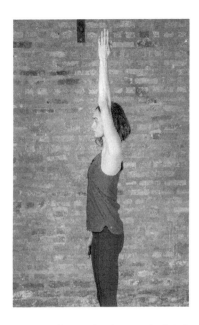

Closing angle joint binding or pinch is indicative of a capsular restriction and should be cleared prior to progressing into the particular motion. Notice in the picture above her ability to raise the arm up to 180° without compensation, or dependency on other regions to achieve the motion.

The important question to ask is: WHY is the capsule limited? Clinically, I've correlated this closing angle pain with an anterior sitting humeral head in the glenoid fossa. If the head already sits anterior, motions including flexion, abduction and external rotation will be problematic because the bone won't be able to move forward in the joint in order to clear space, resulting in capsular pinching. This impingement could be because a tight joint capsule, tight tissue on the front of the scapula including the pec minor and subscapularis or a number of other potential reasons. This positioning can be correlated to a number of issues common among those with posterior shoulder pain, including muscular restrictions, poor posture, joint restrictions and altered length tension relationships.

KEY CONCEPT: The posterior shoulder complex is related fascially to a number of different highways, including the Posterior Flexibility Highway and Posterior X line. For throwers and swing sport participants particularly, always make sure to check the opposite hip into internal rotation.

Throwers and those playing swing sports (including racquet, stick or otherwise) often demonstrate an inability to fully internally rotate and flex the hip, results in overworking to the posterior shoulder to decelerate the arm at follow through, which would otherwise be decelerated by the opposite hip.

This lack of hip internal rotation also may affect the low back on the limited hip side because the lumbar spine, which isn't designed for a lot of rotation, is forced to make up the difference for the hip.

What is the position of the humeral head in the glenoid fossa?

Integrated exercises emphasizing the posterior shoulder include:

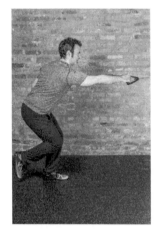

Posterior X squat to row start (with or without toe touch support)

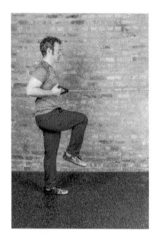

Posterior X squat to row end

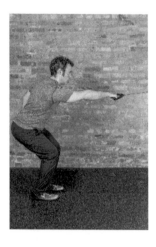

Posterior X squat to row start (regression and with bilateral LE support)

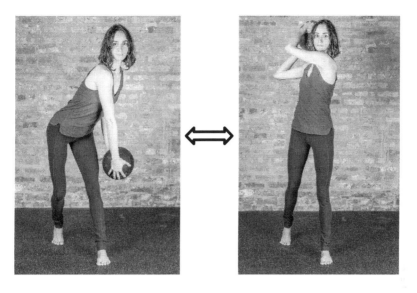

Rotational wood chops are excellent for training both the Anterior & Posterior X lines. Emphasis sin on keeping a 'long spine' and rotating from the pelvis. Remember, where the pelvis goes, the low back will follow. This is also a good movement to train and teach to those with low back pain or difficulty with lifting mechanics. It can be regressed or progressed in a variety of ways. If difficult to perform, check hip flexion/adduction/Internal rotation of the hip, and also thoracic mobility into type 1 & 2 motion.

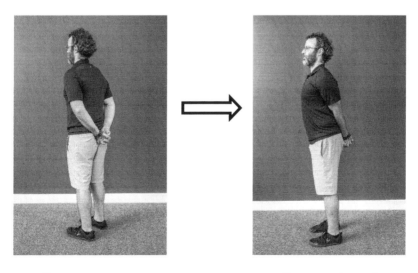

Chest expansion, start   Chest expansion, end

Frozen Shoulder

Adhesive capsulitis is rare in patients younger than 40 and more common in sedentary workers than laborers, particularly women. Remember a joint is defined as space between bones, and around the heads of the two bones is the equivalent of saran wrap. This tissue is the deepest layer of connective tissue and surrounds the heads of the bones, considered the joint capsule. The capsule wraps the heads of the bones in 360 degrees to allow the correct amount of roll, slide and glide of one bone against the other. Adhesive capsulitis occurs for various reasons, sometimes of known origin and often times insidiously, where the capsule becomes tight and bound down and altering proper humeral-scapulothoracic motion to occur. Hammer (2009) describes a progressive fibrous proliferation that restricts mostly lateral rotation. They describe a fibrosis of the articular capsule and the rotator cuff tendons.

It's important to remember that the shoulder is a *complex* and made up of 4 joints. While typically the limitation is seen in the glenohumeral joint, more often than not it there is enough motion in the GH joint, however the true limitation is between the scapula, thorax and the axillary musculature that is found in that space. Ensuring proper motion of the scapula on the thorax, and that the thoracic spine has as much motion as possible is of utmost benefit. Ensuring the scapula has as many decrees of in all direction is imperative. In addition, clinically I've noticed those with this pathology typically have difficulty diaphragmatically breathing. While ensuring the shoulder complex has adequate mobility, breathing and decreasing a sympathetic state must also be considered.

While passive stretching of the glenohumeral joint is helpful to increase Range of Motion (ROM) with adhesive capsulitis, increasing hip and thoracic motion is also helpful. Mobilizing the shoulder while the hips are being authentically lengthened also allows for greater shoulder mobility.

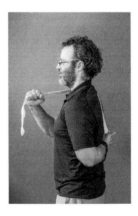

Posterior shoulder stretch with posterior humeral head glide

Forearm & Elbow Pain: Anatomy Overview

Like most other body parts, when the elbow hurts it isn't the elbow's fault. The site of the pain isn't the cause of the pain, unless it is a crush injury (think a piano falling on your head while walking down the street). The elbow is an extension of the shoulder, scapula, and thoracic spine, and limited motion here can result in increased stress to the distal areas, creating intramuscular tender points and adhesions. These can easily be dealt with by incorporating soft tissue modalities and the correct movement patterns that are geared towards preserving joint mobility. The medial and lateral forearm and elbow muscles are related to different lines of the body, including the spiral lines and functional arm lines and should be considered for treatment and movement patterns.

Lateral Forearm Pain/ Lateral Epicondylitis= Tennis Elbow

Lateral Epicondylitis, also called tennis elbow, is a garbage bucket term summating many different pathologies, and so differentiation as to WHY the lateral elbow is hurting is critical. In addition to being soft tissue in nature, other diagnosis that are associated with this part of the body include osteoarthritis, tenosynovitis, nerve compression from a variety of causes including radial nerve entrapment, ulnar neuropathy and median nerve compression (aka, carpal tunnel syndrome).

Lateral epicondylitis is a general term that means the muscles that attach to or around the lateral epicondyle, or outside of the elbow are in some sort of inflammatory cycle. These muscles include attachments of the wrist and hand extensors at the top and distally to various hand bones, in addition to the brachioradialis which attaches to the distal shaft of the humerus above the elbow and distally to the styloid process of the radius. The integrated function of the extensor muscles is to control wrist flexion and stabilize for the finger flexors when they are used to grasp, while the brachioradialis primarily assists in controlling forearm flexion and rotation motions, such as unscrewing a lid.

In the cases of lateral epicondylitis, traditionally treated by rubbing on the irritated tissue surrounding the lateral epicondyle combined with stretching and strengthening the wrist extensors. At times this treatment option works, but many times progress isn't seen because the wrist extensors, based on length tension relationships, tend to be less connected to the nervous system and therefore treatment approach must also change. I've found that often times, the lateral wrist extensor tissue's neural drive lessened, demonstrated by a weak muscle test. When this is the case, stretching and soft tissue work to the wrist extensor tissue will lessen the neural drive even more, and can potentially exacerbate the situation. I've found that often times that balancing out the length tension relationship between the tissue on both sides of the elbow and wrist allows a more even distribution of forces become more symmetrical two sides of the elbow. When this happens, there will be a greater connection of the extensors to the nervous system and consequently a better ability to engage that tissue.

KEY CONCEPT: Important points to consider in resolving lateral elbow pain is that fascially it is an extension of the muscles that attach to the shoulder blade. These include the triceps & parascapular muscles, and kinetically are a part of many fascial highway connections, including the lateral line and posterior X line.

Areas of the body to check to ensure have enough motion, (so the lateral elbow muscles don't have to move too much) include the thoracic spine and opposite hip. If either of those areas aren't able to move enough, in order to decelerate a swing the lateral elbow muscles (if not the posterior shoulder) are forced to do too much to decelerate the motion. In addition, ensuring the proper length of the wrist flexors and intrinsic muscles of the hand is also important, and if not working properly often coincide with overactive wrist extensors.

Are the wrist flexors tight, creating asymmetry between flexors and extensors?

Does client have full supination and pronation?

What is the resting position of the hands? They should be next to the body, thumbs pointing forward and hands facing each other, not in front of the body.

Motions and exercise to include are:

Lateral chain exercises that emphasize frontal plane hip and thoracic spine mobility, where the wrist flexors can be lengthened in an integrated fashion has proven to be helpful in minimizing elbow pain.

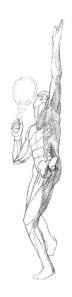

Lateral Flexibility Highway

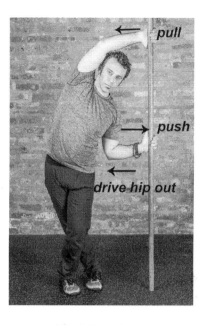

Lateral flexibility highway stretch
utilizing principles of tensegrity

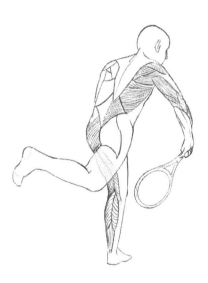

Posterior X Flexibility Highway

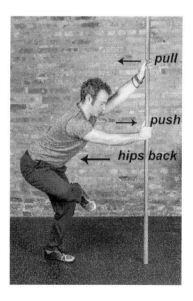

Posterior X Stretch utilizing principles of tensegrity

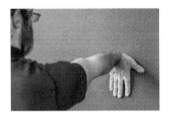 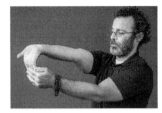 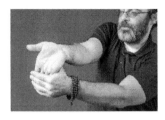

Wrist flexor stretch against wall

Wrist flexor stretch without wall

Wrist flexor stretch with compensation. Notice elevated shoulder, side bending in spine and decreased supination

---

Medial Forearm Pain/ Golfers Elbow

Medial epicondylitis, also known as golfer's elbow, is inflammation of the tissue attaching to the medial portion of the humeral epicondyle. Like other issues that arise in the body, the medial epicondyle can be a point of irritation and develop tender points. These can be relieved with soft tissue work, especially if the overall musculature around the elbow and upper extremity is out of balance. Like other areas of the body, the tissue that attaches into the medial forearm is part of a larger fascial organization, including the anterior X highway, connecting the front of the arm and chest to the opposite hip, through the core on a diagonal. In addition, I've found that often times grip strength is an issue, and so the medial elbow/wrist tissue works too hard to compensate.

Clinically when someone presents with this medial elbow pain I think about the chain reactions that occur, and the tissue that tends to lengthen together to control forces. Remember, most times the site of the pain isn't the cause of the pain. My experience is that medial elbow tissue irritation is often times associated with poor posture and in swing sport athletes often combined with an inability of the spine to lengthen into side bending and rotating towards the area that is injured.

Increasing the length and strength of the same side lat and length of the same side pec minor can often decrease the stress to the medial elbow tissue, and that can be accomplished with an Anterior X stretch. This can be done via a same side rotational lunge w/ a rotational arm reach to emphasize the end range load to the wrist flexors.

KEY CONCEPT: Check thoracic rotation & side bending towards the side of limitation.

Check Anterior X motions

Grip strength

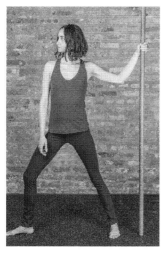

PROGRESSION ➡

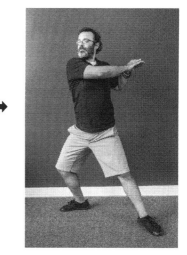

Same-side rotational lunge Right
Leg right 135° holding onto post

Same-side rotational lunge right
leg right 135°

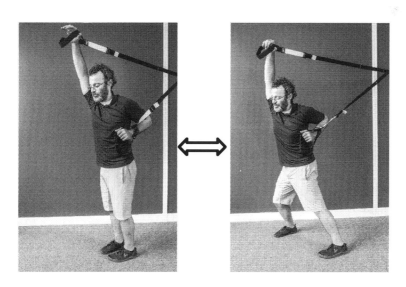

Suspension strap type two thoracic
motion lunge with emphasis on
frontal plane start

Suspension strap type two thoracic
motion lunge with emphasis on
frontal plane end

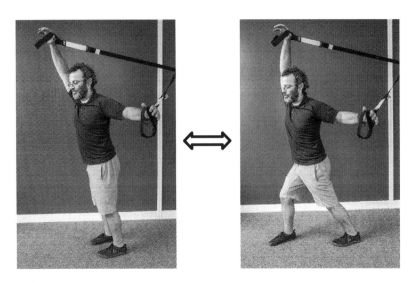

Suspension strap type two thoracic motion lunge with emphasis on transverse plane start

Suspension strap type two thoracic motion lunge with emphasis on transverse plane end

Additional Reading List:

Osar, Evan. Corrective Exercise Solutions to Common Shoulder and Hip Dysfunction

Page, Phillip, Clare C. Frank, and Robert Lardner. Assessment and Treatment of Muscle Imbalance: The Janda Approach.

Gray, G. Functional Video Digest Series. Vol. 1.3 The Most ability Shoulder: Every Which Way but Loose, Vol 4.2 Functional Manual Reaction: The Shoulder

Iyengar, B. K. Light on yoga: Yoga dipika

Wolf, Chuck, DVD. Functional Integrated Shoulder Training

Desikachar, T. K. The heart of yoga: Developing a personal practice. Rochester, VT: Inner Traditions International.

Isaacs, E. R., Bookhout, M. R., & Bourdillon, J. F. (2002). Bourdillon's spinal manipulation.

CHAPTER 10

Exercise Library

This movement glossary is designed as an adjunct to the bulk of the text, and by no means is an extensive library. Rather, it's a more in-depth description of some of the movements mentioned that have been of useful to me in my movement practices. It purposefully does not include any "core" or "breathing" exercises because there are so many and an entire book have and could be written about it. The movements described here are nothing more than a piece of a puzzle, and based on a thought process of a biopsychosocial conscious to unconscious spectrum. Any and all of the movements can be regressed and progressed many ways. Of course, breathing should be considered with all movements, and if the breath is held during motion, it likely means they're past the neurological threshold. For those that do clench their jaws and hold their breath, or don't breathe fluid and rhythmically, oftentimes performing the movement mouth open provides an additional training variable can be difficult for those with jaw dysfunction.

On the spectrum of movement, these exercises range from increasing motor patterning, such as isolated toe movements, which are designed bring awareness to the lack of ability to and also to create space in the motor cortex. Other exercises are geared towards lengthening and loading entire chains of tissue together in order to control a specific motion, such as a lunge with a reach (or a wood chop) which can mimic the first transformational zone of lifting up a box at ground height. There are also movements that isolate out specific body parts within an integrated movement, such as the suspension strap type two lunges or child's pose with breathing, designed to both enhance diaphragmatic excursion and increase thoracic extension.

1st Toe extension

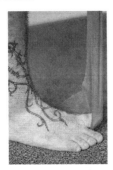 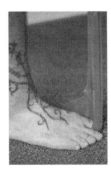

- Sitting in a chair with feet firmly placed under knees
- Raise (extend) 1st Toe without moving toes 2-5
  - Compensation is to flex the proximal interphalangeal joints, or extend the distal interphalangeal joints
- Hold for 6 count
- Return to starting position
  - Regressions include: extending all toes at once, and placing toes 2-5 down (either together or 5,4,3,2), keeping the 1st toe extended
  - Progressions include standing and loading the toes with tband

2-5 Toe extension

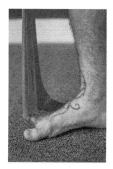 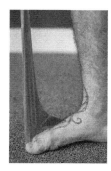

- Sitting in a chair with feet firmly placed under knees
- Raise (extend) toes 2-5 without moving 1st toe
  - Compensation is to flex the first toe (or sometimes extend) or to dorsiflex the ankle
- Hold for 6 count
- Return to starting position
  - Regressions include extending all toes at once, and placing 1st toe down, keeping 2-5 extended
  - Progressions include standing or loading 1st toe w/ tband

Toe intrinsic strength w/ tband

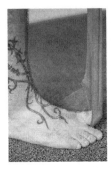 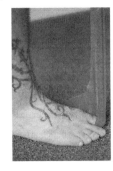 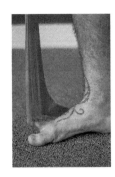 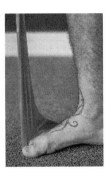

- Place theraband under foot, wrapping either the 1st toe, or toes 2-5
- Tension band w/ toe(s) passively taken into extension
- Pull toes down towards floor, using proximal interphalangeal joint(s)
  - A common compensation is to extend the distal interphalangeal joints with flexion of the proximal interphalangeal joints
- 1-3 sets 10-20 reps, emphasizing form rather than numbers

Chest expansion

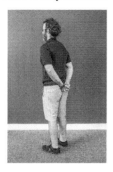 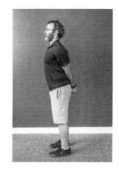 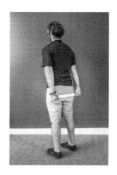 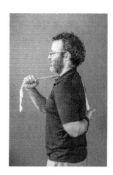

- Stand straight, feet parallel, shoulder width apart.
- Interlace fingers behind you
  - ○ Regression is holding a strap or towel
- Straighten arms and "reach for heels" while putting the top of the head on the ceiling
- Energetically lengthen and pull clavicles laterally expand shoulders
- Progression: forward fold, pulling hands up and over the body.

Child's pose with Type 2 Thoracic Spine (side bending/rotation to same side)

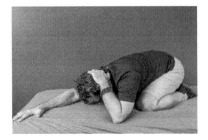 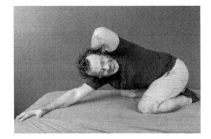

- Kneel on floor, touch toes together and sit on heels, & separate knees as wide as hips
- Exhale and lay your chest between your thighs. Widen the back of your pelvis and narrow the ASIS down onto the inner thighs.
- Reach hands overhead to shoulder are flexed (there should be no pinching in the closing angle of the shoulders)
- Spider crawl hands to the left, so the right hand is just to the left of midline. Take left hand and place behind the neck, with left elbow pointed down towards floor.
- With a long slow inhale (ideally through the nose), raise the left elbow up towards the ceiling, attempting to look at the ceiling under the left armpit
- With a long, slow exhale, return to the starting position
- The breath should last slightly longer than the movement

Down dog

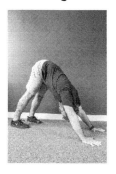 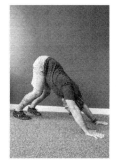 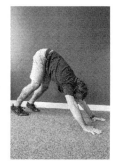 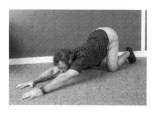

- From table top position (hands & knees), make sure knees are directly below hips and hands are slightly forward of the shoulders. Spread palms with middle finger pointed forward.
- Lift knees away from floor, pushing through hands and lifting the pelvis & ischial tuberosity up and towards the ceiling with knees slightly flexed and heels off the ground. The arms should be flexed and externally rotated, with a long neck.
- Breathe deeply, ideally through the nose, with long, slow exhales.
- Straighten knees, but don't' lock them and drop the heels to the ground.
- Envision keeping the pelvis and rib cage stacked over each other, relative to the position the body is in
- Attempt to create as much distance between the hands and the tailbone as possible, keeping proper alignment.
  - Down dog can be regressed by bending the knees and lifting the heels towards the ceiling. However optimal alignment of the spine and rib cage aligned over the pelvis is important.
- Scapula's should be down the spine, with a long neck in the front, back and sides.
- Down dog, or Adho Mukha Svanasana is a post of the Sun Salutation sequence in yoga.
- This movement is one I use, while interchanging between a plank and down dog, emphasizing breath and cuing to maintain a neutral spine.

Lunge

Lunging is a great movement for virtually all populations because of the ease of regression & progression. A lunge is a motion that moves the body away from midline via a step (however big), followed by a return to the starting position. This movement should look clean, fluid and rhythmical. While others may define it differently, to me these are the keys to an effective lunge. A lunge is a great assessment tool because they can easily mimic and accentuate the motions of an activity. It also transfers into an exercise or stretch performed at home, and can be regressed and progressed depending on the thresholds of the individual. Strategies of progression/regression include speed, velocity and amplitude, or how fast, how far to step, and how deep into a motion. Strategies of regression include simple weight shifts in any plane of motion. While a weight shift mimics the front foot in gait, it's less authentic than taking a step because a step creates a bottom-up motion into the front foot, while a weight shift causes a top-down motion into the foot. In addition, arm reaches combined with visual points can create expected specific reactions. As I often say, if you know what should happen when you drive someone in space, you can see if it happens or not, and if it doesn't happen, ask Why!

The Gray Institute defines various types of lunges, which are described below. In short, there are 6 main vectors in which to lunge or reach. They are anterior/posterior in the sagittal plane, same-side lateral/opposite-side lateral in the frontal plane, and same-side rotational/opposite-side rotational in the transverse plane, and can be combined infinitely.

KEY CONCEPT: A lunge should be clean, fluid, and rhythmical and is a great assessment tool. If you know what should happen, you can check to see if it is happening.

Reaches

Reaches are a phenomenal tool to be able to create a reaction in another body part. A reach is simply using a body part and moving it in space at a particular angle, horizontal distance, and verticality. As we've mentioned in this text, if you know what should happen reaching to a particular place in space, you can see if it happens or not. Reaches can be used to "tweak in" or "tweak out" a body part. For example, when performing a common sagittal plane, or forward lunge, reaching at a verticality of knee height versus shoulder height will "tweak in" the gluteus complex in the sagittal plane, compared with reaching at shoulder height with the lunge. Another example is during the same forward lunge, rotating the arms into the stepping leg, (with a right leg forward lunge, the arms rotate to the right), "tweaks in" the glutes in the transverse plane, and rotating the arms away from the stepping foot, or arms rotating left with a right leg forward lunge "tweaks out" the gluteus complex in the transverse plane.

The variables with reaches include, speed, horizontal distance (i.e. how far in front of the knee) and verticality (reaching at knee vs. shoulder height). Common reaches include forward, same side, side-reach, and same side rotational reach, similar to a common lunge, while uncommon reaches include overhead, opposite side, side-reach and an opposite side rotational reach.

KEY POINT:

Common reach & lunge: with pictures

      Anterior/Forward

      Same-side side

      Same-side rotational

Uncommon reach & lunge

      Posterior/Overhead

      Opposite-side side

      Opposite -side rotational

Common lunges

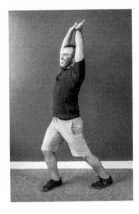
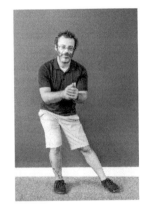
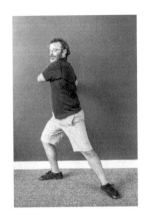

Anterior   Same-side lateral   Same-side rotational

- **Anterior**
    - From starting position, lunge forward to position where there is rhythm and fluidity during the transition from the eccentric lengthening into the concentric shortening.
    - Return to start
    - *Be sure to strike with heel if mimicking gait.*
    - *Think synchronous dissociation with the motion. Is it being synchronously dissociated? Would shortening, or altering the angle/speed/distance of the movement make it so?*
    - With or without common or uncommon reaches
- **Same-side lateral**
    - From starting position, to comfortable step 90° to the same side
    - The emphasis of the movement should be the translation of the pelvis out past the knee and foot.
        - A verbal cue that helps is to "shine" the flashlight in the belly button in front of the *trail leg (left if lunging right) toes.* This ensures that there is both translation and rotation of the pelvis.
    - The emphasis of the motion is fluidity and rhythm. Compensations often include the tibia and femur moving laterally at the same time. There needs to be dissociation in order for the hip to feel the transformational zone consistent with the first zone of gait, which is knee flexion/abduction/internal

rotation and hip flexion/adduction/internal rotation. Be sure there is synchronous dissociation

  ○ With or without common or uncommon reaches

● Same-side rotational

  ○ From starting position, rotate right leg to the right at the appropriate vector anywhere from R-90°-R180°, depending on objective of lunge

    ■ Upon the foot hitting the ground, and at the end of the load into the motion, the pelvis should be squared to the direction of the foot, unless there is a reason not to (IE, you're choosing to bypass the motion of the foot complex by landing into the lunge in an internally rotated foot position, in order to create a specific motion at the hip that wouldn't otherwise be attained because of the position of the foot. This would be a choice as a movement option for a foot dysfunction that contributes to a hip pain, and in conjunction with an exercise addressing the reason why the foot isn't able to load into pronation, creating the proper rear-foot and tibial motion.

  ○ Return to starting position, with emphasis on, fluidity and rhythm the same speed in and out.

  ○ With or without common and uncommon reaches

*note the difference between a frontal plane and rotational lunge is classified relative to the direction the stepping foot faces upon the foot hitting the ground. A same side 90° lunge can be a frontal plane or a transverse plane lunge, depending on the direction the stepping foot is facing. For example, a frontal plane lunge to same-side 90° will have the toes facing forward, stepping to 90° right, but pointed to 0° (or straight ahead); whereas a same-side 90° lunge would be classified as a rotational lunge is the stepping foot (right foot) is pointed towards the 90° vector, or the toe facing "3" on a clock, on a rotational lunge. Forward is relative to the direction of the stepping foot. Therefore in the first example of a frontal plane 90° lunge the chest pointed forward would be pointed 'straight ahead' toward the zero degree vector. While the chest/torso would be pointed 90° to the right w/ a transverse plane lunge.

Uncommon lunge

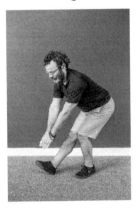
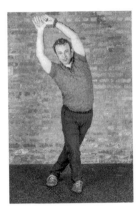
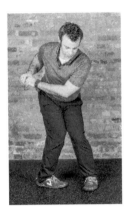

Posterior Lunge   Opposite-side side lunge   Opposite-side rotational lunge

- Posterior Lunge
  - Front standing position, step backwards with right leg and sit hips "back into chair", straightening front (left) knee through motion
    - I describe this motion as an 'active hamstring stretch'
  - Only step as far as you can without having to pause at the bottom of the motion, and return to start
  - Emphasis is on distance and being fluid and rhythmical during exercise.
  - With or without common or uncommon lunges
- Opposite-side side lunge
  - From starting position, right leg steps/lunges to left, across body, with right foot landing pointed at zero degree vector (forward)
  - Load into the motion with fluidity and rhythm.
    - Chest should be pointed forward in direction of right foot
  - Return to starting position
  - With or without common or uncommon lunges
- Opposite-side rotational lunge
  - From starting position, right leg rotates left with right foot landing with toes facing left 90 degrees with chest facing left 90 degrees in direction of right toes
  - Only step as far as possible without having to pause at the bottom of the motion, emphasizing speed, fluidity and rhythm.
  - return to starting position
  - With or without common or uncommon reaches.

Balance to lunge

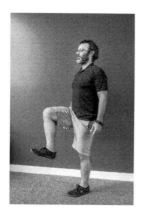 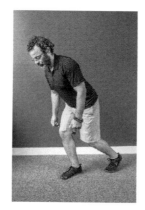 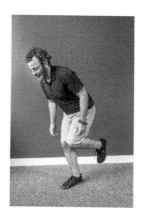

- Starting in single leg balance position
  - ○ Modified by toe touch support or hand touch support at wall
- Perform common or uncommon lunge and return to starting position, emphasizing stopping completely at 'top' or start of motion before performing another repetition
- Common or uncommon lunges
- With or without common or uncommon reaches

Lateral flexibility highway stretch

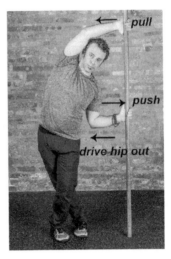

This stretch takes advantage of the principles of tensegrity, by pushing (compressing) and pulling (tensioning) the system.

- Standing next to door or pole, with Right shoulder closest
- Cross inside leg (Right leg) over outside leg (left leg)
- Take outside hand (left hand) up overhead and grab the pole
    - Right hand goes to door at roughly waist height, or where desired for specificity in stretch with the lateral line
- Pull with top (left) hand, push with the bottom (right) hand

Posterior X:

The posterior X highway is one that's incorporated into my practice frequently. I think about movements being progressed along a spectrum, from static to dynamic. A stretch that incorporates the posterior shoulder muscles on one side and the posterior hip muscles on the other can be lengthened and strengthened together from a position and also through a motion. For example, with the left leg forward in a "lunging" position with a post to the outside of the left shoulder, if the right arm reaches across the body and grabs the post, the right posterior shoulder/lat, along with the left posterior hip muscles are being lengthened together. In this instance, if the right hand pulls, and the left hand pushes, the posterior X is being tensioned together, utilizing the principles of tensegrity. That same static movement can be made more dynamic first by driving the pelvis in three planes of motion (forward/back, side/side, rotation) to begin to drive motion into the tissue and make it lengthen together. From the same position, if the left leg performs a forward step/lunge, the left lengthens dynamically along with the right posterior shoulder and latissimus. Taking the same tissue, and lengthening it together even more dynamically would involve the left leg performing a lunge with the right hand reaching across the body, somewhere around the knee (or above/below depending on the specificity of the load).

I like strengthen the para-scapular muscles involved in isolated scapular retraction with the opposite gluteus complex concurrently concentrically shortening. Like the above described stretch, this 'strengthening' motion can also be progressed or regressed, depending on the needs of the individual. Below are described squat to pulls, step to pulls, balance w/ rows, and other exercises that incorporate the opposite hip and shoulder.

Posterior X stretch

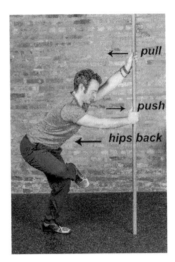

- Standing next to (or in front of) a door or something to grab onto.
- Place hands at shoulder (or where is appropriate for the individual) with left hand above right hand.
- Cross right ankle over left knee (or place right foot on chair or step)
- While holding post, sit back into chair, so pelvis drops down and back and the right hip is flexed, and externally rotated.
- Pull with left (top) hand, push with right (bottom) hand.
    - O Specificity to the stretch can be attained by moving pushing hand up or down the post, depending on where the location in the limitation in the chain.

Squat to Press Section

LWE squat to triplane OH press

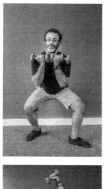 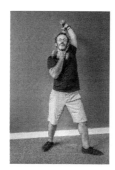 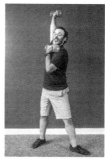 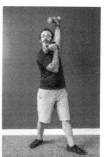

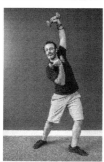 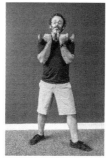 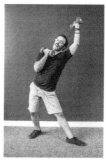 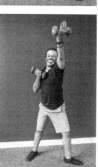

LWE stands for left leg forward in the sagittal plane, "L", feet wider than shoulder width apart in the frontal planes "W", and feet externally rotated in the transverse plane "E". This nomenclature is developed by the Gray Institute. It is a very smart way to describe starting motions and also positions, and can describe the sequence of a movement.

- With left leg forward, feet wider than shoulder apart, both feet externally rotated
- Begin with dumbbells in racked, or bottom position, with palms in front of, and facing shoulders
- Squat with hands in racked position
- Stand and press one hand overhead
    - Note, there are 6 vectors to reach to, overhead anterior/posterior, overhead same side lateral, overhead opposite side lateral, overhead same side rotational, overhead opposite side rotational. See pictures.
- Return to starting position

Post X Single Leg squat to pull

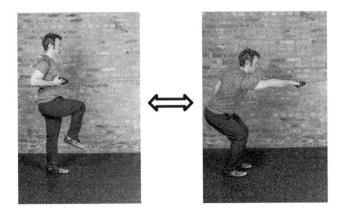

- ● Right hand holding cable
- ● Squat on left leg w/ right leg reaching behind & right arm reaching towards cable
    - ○ This eccentrically lengthens the opposite posterior shoulder and hip
- ● Stand and pull
    - ○ Bringing right leg to balance position or right leg to toe touch support
- ● Return to starting position

Note that this movement can be progressed or regressed based on the amount of support she needs to keep a steady and balanced position

Post X rotational step w/ shoulder ER

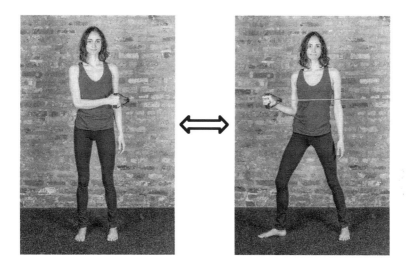

- Start in squat (or stance with knees flexed)
- Right hand holding cable/band on vector of forward to left 90'
- Load further into motion (squat)
- Stand and externally rotate
  - ○ Squat to stand w/ external rotation of left hip and also right shoulder external rotation

Wood chop knee to shoulder

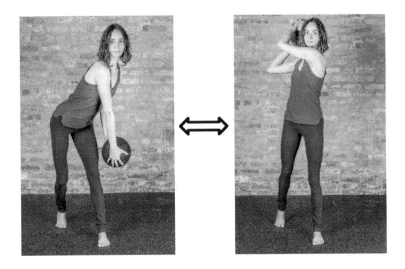

- Stand tall and hold medicine ball with both hands at chest height
- Squat down, and with a long spine, bring the ball to the outside of the knee
  - Be sure to pivot and move from the hips, not the low back or spine.
- Stand and twist the torso as far as possible in the opposite direction, bringing the ball up and above your opposite shoulder.
- Return ball to knee
- Momentum is your friend! Remember, the rotational plane is parallel with gravity, and therefore it's pure muscle action to control this motion.
- Move from the pelvis with a long spine!
  - Don't squat down to bring the ball lower, and don't flex through the spine!

Wallbanger/Rotational Squat

The following description is adapted from Chuck Wolf's description of a wallbanger. I learned this exercise from Chuck early in my career, and it's been a go to ever since a wallbanger is essentially a rotational squat. The cue of shine the flashlight in your bellybutton is most important with this exercise, because where the pelvis goes, the low back will follow. If the pelvis is limited in the frontal or transverse planes, often times there will not be enough pelvic rotation, resulting in too much motion through the lumbar spine, particularly at L4-L5 and L5-S1 spine levels. This is an effective movement pattern for those with foot, knee, hip and low back pain. One reason I like it is because it gets the foot, knee and hip to work together and mimic what they would do and when they would do it.

The following describes the movement for the RIGHT HIP.

- Stand about 4-6 inches off the wall, in athletic position & STAND TALL! This is the starting position.
- Squat and rotate away from the wall, whining the flashlight in the belly button in front of the left foot
- Be sure to translate the pelvis lateral to the knee and foot, and tap the lateral hip into the wall and return to starting position.
- A great cue is to squish a bug under the right big toe and inside of the medial border of the calcaneus. This is a cue I learned from a fantastic book called *Harvey Pennicks Little Red Book: Lessons and Teaching from a Lifetime in Golf.*
  - Letting the big toe come up and the weight to the lateral side of the foot is a huge biomechanical leak. If the foot doesn't do what it needs to do, when it needs to do it, neither will the hip.

Self-Myofascial Release Section

Releases are designed to "pin-and-stretch" tissue in order to improve the ability of the layers of tissue to glide past each other. The following are regions that clinically I've found to be beneficial.

SMR adductor:

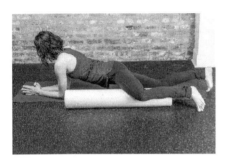 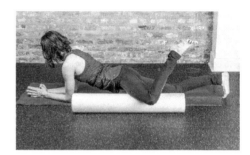

- Starting in a plank position, lower onto foam roll
  - (the foam roll is parallel to the body)
- Bend the working leg to the side, placing the medial thigh onto the roll.
- Keep non-working leg straight
- With core engaged, roll from the knee <> pelvis.
- When tender spot found, perform deep nasal breaths with long, slow exhales
- Lift ankle (of bend knee) toward the ceiling x3 repetitions before moving on
- Pick 1-2 spot per pass to stop and move the leg on. On next pass, pick the same or different spots

SMR Calf

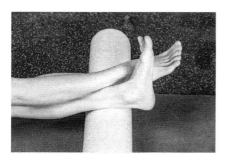 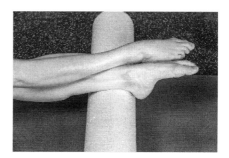

- Sit on ground in 'long sit' position.
- Foam roll should be placed on calcaneus
- Sit with hands behind the body for support
- Place the non-working foot on the shin, directly above the foam roll for added compression
- Roll from ankle<>knee
- When tender spot found, perform deep nasal breaths with long, slow exhales
- Over tender spot, perform ankle dorsiflexion-plantar flexion x 3, roll tibia left-right x 3, then perform ankle circles in each direction x 3

SMR Calf with 2 Balls

- Position working leg bent forward, with non-working leg extended out to the side or into a hurdler's position
  - ○ 90/90 hip position is the easiest, however not everyone can attain this position
- Place one ball between ground and lateral tibia, where the posterior musculature intersects with the lateral musculature, and one ball directly over the bottom ball, between the medial tibia, where the posterior musculature intersects with the medial muscles (see picture for set up)
- Keep torso elevated, and use opposite hand for additional support.
- When tender spot is found, perform deep nasal breaths with long, slow exhales
- Over tender spot, compress top ball towards bottom ball while plantar flexing,>dorsiflexing, next pivot top ball in circular motion clockwise and counterclockwise
- Explore areas between medial malleoli and medial knee

SMR Anterior Chest/Pec Minor:

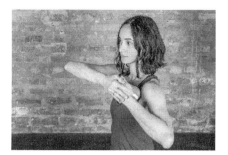 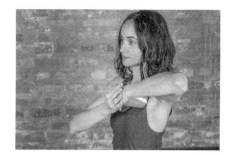

- To identify landmark, front of shoulder towards the naval
- Position ball under heel of hand, with other hand placed on top, or use a yoga block for additional compression and better angle
- Stand/Sit straight with torso elevated
- Scan for tender spot, when found perform deep nasal breaths with long, slow exhales
- With elbows wide, pull one elbow to the ceiling, upwardly rotating the scapula, followed by pulling the elbow towards the ground, downwardly rotating the scapula.
- Ensuring scapular movement during this motion is the key.

SMR Anterior Thigh:

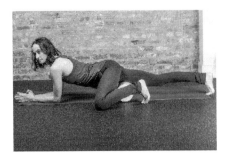 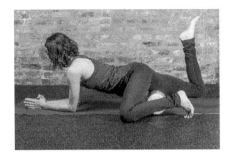

- Starting in plank position, lower onto foam roll w/ roll above the knee cap
  - (the foam roll is perpendicular to the body)
- Bend non-working knee to side, below hip level
- With core engaged, roll in an "army crawl" position from the knee<>pelvis
- When tender spot is found, perform deep nasal breaths with long, slow exhale
- Bend knee x3 repetitions and/or cross friction side<>side at tender spot
- Pick 1-2 spots per pass to stop and bend knee on. On next pass, pick the same or different spots
  - **Variations:**
    - For IT Band/Lateral Quad border:
      - perform a slight turn, in order to angle the roll at the border of the fascial sheath

SMR thoracic:

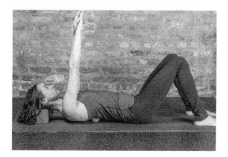 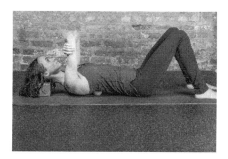

- Identify the bottom of the shoulder blades
- Lay in a supine position with one ball on each side of the spine
- Start by folding hands across chest and 'grabbing opposite elbow'
- "Inch worm" towards the head (the balls will roll towards your pelvis) and back.
- When a 'tender spot' is found, perform deep nasal breaths with long, slow exhales
- Pull elbows side to side

*Note, when rolling balls down into lumbar spine, instead of arm rotations, rotate the knees side to side.

Thoracic spine extension stretch against wall

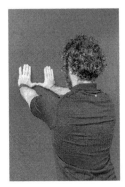 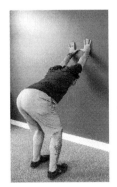 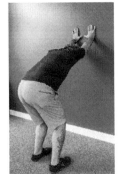 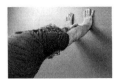

- Standing tall with hands flat on wall, thumbs touching at eye height
- Sit pelvis backwards and down, bending knees and hips backwards
- Keep long spine, with pelvis, ribcage and head aligned

Suspension strap fallout

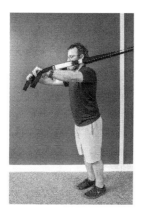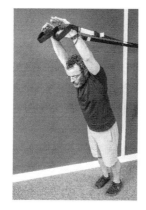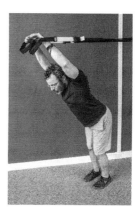

- Begin standing tall with hands at eye height and an engaged core.
- Lean into the straps and move to a plank/push up position. This is the starting position
- Keeping arms straight, lean further into the straps, bringing your body towards the ground while maintaining a neutral spine
  - The arms will flex overhead
  - Make sure not to 'hinge' or 'dump' into the spine, typically at the Cervico-thoracic or thoraco-lumbar junction.
- Pull back by extending arms and maintaining a neutral and engaged spine, and return to the starting position.

Suspension strap intrinsic progression w/ IYT

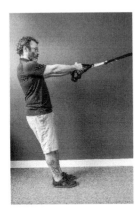 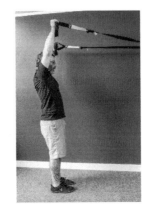 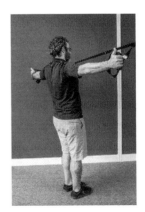

- Stand facing the anchor, feet shoulder width apart
- Hands at approximately mouth height
- Keep "core" engaged, and lean back onto heels until the body forms a diagonal line
- Keeping the spine in neutral and engaged, from the shoulder blades, lift arms into a Y (or T or I), pulling the scapulae down the back and towards middle, keep palms facing
- Return to neutral position w/ neutral spine.

Suspension strap thoracic type 2 lunge

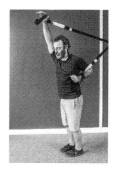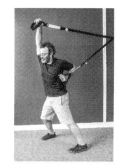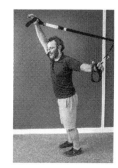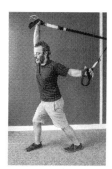

- Begin w/ feet shoulder width apart, toes straight ahead (or in desired starting position)
- Left hand opposite overhead, with tension in strap
- Right hand right rotated, w/ tension in strap.
  - ○ Note: to achieve tension in both straps, make sure to stand in slightly more forward than normal.
  - ○ This starting position places the thoracic spine into a right side bent, right rotated position, or type two motion
- Lunge/step forward at selected vector, with or without alternating steps,
- Return to start position

CHAPTER 11

Conclusion

I n this book, I have described to you, the reader, more or less where I'm headed as a clinician. The following is a summation of the KEY CONCEPT listed in a more formal order, along with some other final thoughts.

The body is one interconnected unit, therefore when one part of the body moves, the whole body responds. Understanding that to effectively stretch the shoulder, incorporating the hips is important because hip extension creates lumbar and thoracic extension, in turn posterior tilting the scapula to allow the humeral head to not impinge on the osseous structure above it. The key is to make sure that the bone that is supposed to be moving faster (or slower) is doing so.

The ability of different layers of tissue to effectively slide and glide past each other is important, and if limited can be palpated as an increased and abrupt tension in a specific region. In addition, often times those that seek therapeutic services tend to be stuck in a negative feedback loop, defined by Merriam Webster as "a reaction that causes a decrease in function, occurring in response to some kind of stimulus. It often causes the output of a system to be lessened, so the feedback tends to stabilize the system." Most people in pain are stuck in a negative feedback loop, which, in my opinion, is interchangeable with an inflammatory cycle and also a cumulative injury cycle.

For those stuck in a negative, or inflammatory feedback loop, I've found that a good strategy to break the loop is to slightly inflame the tissue further while simultaneously working to make behavioral changes. This can be done via a manual intervention or stretching, which brings blood, fluid and awareness to a specific region which creates a better environment for changes to be made. Often times people aren't aware they are stuck in this loop until they're made aware of it. Once they are aware of what they don't' know, the process to integration and behavioral changes can occur.

The challenge is to teach these clients new habits. This involves implementing new behaviors. Those that seek therapy services tend to have a very active sympathetic nervous system, which means learning new behaviors will be more difficult versus those with a parasympathetic dominance. Therefore, one of the primary goals in teaching a new skill set is stimulation of the parasympathetic nervous system because the body create neuroplastic changes, and will learn new tasks easier when in a parasympathetic state. Neuroplasticity is the capacity of the brain to change its structure, and is important for behavior changes.

Our bodies respirate, or perform the subconscious act of taking oxygen in and out of our bodies, approximately 20,000 times per day. So, respiration is subconscious, but breathing is conscious. How many can say they actually consciously breathe? It's been proven that long and slow exhales, particularly through the nose, vibrates the nose hair, called cilia, stimulating parasympathetic response. This in turn, makes it easier to learn new behaviors and tasks.

Movement is defined as a synchronous dissociation of body segments. If two bones move in the same speed at the same direction, the joint doesn't feel anything. In integration, muscles lengthen to control forces presented to the body instead of shortening in isolation to produce a force.

Injury occurs when forces are presented to the body that the body can't handle, typically at the end of the Transformational Zone (TZ). A transformational Zone is defined as the point in time when the body stops loading and begins to unload, and every activity has at least two transformational zones. Three dimensional joint motion is assessed at the TZ, and if the TZ's are known, one can deduce what happens through the motion from one TZ to the other.

Assessing closing angle joint restrictions is a priority before addressing soft tissue restrictions. Motion in the extremities is named for the distal bone moving on a fixed proximal bone, while in the spine, motion is named for the proximal bone moving on a fixed distal bone. When naming three dimensional motion at a joint, there is a process to go through. The first question that must be answered when naming motion at a Transformational Zone is to ask what two bones make up the joint. The second is to ask if the bones are moving in the same or opposite direction around each axis in each plane of motion, and the third question to ask is which bone is moving faster, the top or bottom bone.

Motion is driven into the system that the body must control. A Driver is defined as a way to create a reaction, and a physical driver is defined as a way to subconsciously create a reaction in another body part. Physical drivers are found all over the body, and can include the hand, foot, pelvis, knee, and eyes, which Gary Gray calls one of the most powerful drivers. The eyes, and also the bottom of the feet, are going to remain horizontal to the ground. Therefore, if there is an eye dysfunction, the eyes will remain horizontal while the body moves around a fixed head to compensate, often resulting in cervical spine dysfunction. A top down driver implies that the top bones move in the direction faster than the bottom bones; and a bottom up driver implies the bottom bones move in a direction faster than the top bones. Motion in the extremities is named for how the distal bone moving on a fixed proximal bone; while motion in the extremities is named for how the proximal bone moves on a fixed distal bone. For example, the first TZ is a bottom up motion into the system, because the foot hits the ground first and causes motion above, while the second TZ in gait is a top down motion because the back femur moves in response to the pelvis moving above it.

Remember that naming three dimensional movement can be a challenging process, especially as these strategies are beginning to be incorporated into your work. If you have trouble finding why, make sure to check the foot, hip and thoracic spine; as these are often times the areas that don't do enough, forcing the areas above and below to do too much. A suggestion is to pick a few movements, perhaps the flexibility highways, and have all your clients go through the movements, if appropriate. Only through repetition and continued effort to learn new information will it become an effective part of your repertoire. In addition, my hope is that the recognition of this information powerfully affects people will be a reason for YOU to keep learning and expanding as a movement practitioner.

With prescription of specific movements each session, continual evaluation and updates to programs are necessary. This ensures each session is individualized based on the person in front of you that day, and this can be easily accomplished recognizing that the test is the exercise, and the exercise is the test.

I feel fortunate to love what I do, and continually feel the need to add to my toolbox. The disciplines of integrated motion and motor control insight (muscle testing) are powerful modalities individually, and I believe I'm a better clinician because I combine these modalities. My plan is to continue refining my movement understanding, evaluation skills and therapeutic prescription, which will always be something I do. I'm also intent on refining my muscle testing skills in order to be more efficient. To that end, my upcoming studies will be advanced courses in muscle testing, as well as an extremity adjustment course later this year, taught by Chiropractor Dan McClure. I'm also very interested in pain sciences and hope to take a course taught by Lorimer Moseley because his writings and video's on pain science are top notch, and I also hope to learn from Dr. Andreo Spina more in the future. Finally, a course that's definitely on my list is Functional Neuro-Orthopedic Rehabilitation (FNOR), however this is more of a long term goal, as the FNOR program is multi-month and quite intensive.

In conclusion, what's exciting for me is that the more I understand, the more questions I have. I hope to continue working to synthesize my process in order to find "the answer" to underlying pain and dysfunction. While I recognize there isn't "one answer", my goal is to continue refining and enhancing my skills so that I can best serve those with whom I work.

This text has been a great exercise for me, and has furthered my understanding on all these topics. My assumption is that you, the reader, also desire to better yourself, and I believe if you've read this far, it's likely the case. I encourage you to learn directly from those who have influenced me, and also check online for further work on synthesizing different movement modalities. I already recognize areas to flesh out further and enhance, as well as other topics to write, synthesize and learn about.

Finally, if what I've discussed here has sparked your interest, I encourage you to check out some of my other offerings, including in person and online courses and videos on different movement, bodywork, and motor control related topics. Currently, my favorite courses to teach include a 2 day course called "Improving Fascial Highways: A Perspective on Integrated Motion & Motor Control", and also body part specific one day courses including "Where Does the Low Back Go When It Goes out? The Key's to a No Whine Lumbar Spine" and "What Every Giraffe Knows that We Don't; The Key's to a No Whine Cervical Spine". I also teach Functional Movement Techniques (FMT) courses on behalf of Rocktape, which are incredibly fun to teach. The FMT courses are really movement courses within the context of applying adhesive elastic tape. To go further in depth, consider purchasing the 2 day course, which is an adjunct to this book and offers more in depth information about all topics discussed.

All of this and more can be found online at www.biomechanicaldetective.com

Bibliography

Barral, J. P., and Pierre Mercier. *Visceral Manipulation*. Seattle: Eastland, 2005. Print.

Billis, Evdokia V., Christopher J. Mccarthy, and Jacqueline A. Oldham. "Subclassification of Low Back Pain: A Cross-country Comparison." *European Spine Journal Eur Spine J* 16.7 (2007): 865-79. Web.

Bordoni, Bruno, and Emiliano Zanier. "Skin, Fascias, and Scars: Symptoms and Systemic Connections." *Journal of Multidisciplinary Healthcare JMDH* (2013): 11. Web.

Bove GM, Chapelle SL. Visceral mobilization can lyse and prevent post-surgical adhesions. Journal of Bodywork and Movement Therapies, 16, 76-82, 2012 doi: 10.1016/j.jbmt.2011.02.004

Bove, G. M., Chapelle, S. L., Boyle, E., Mokler, D. J., & Hartvigsen, J. (2016). A Novel Method for Evaluating Postoperative Adhesions in Rats. Journal of Investigative Surgery, 1-7.

Bove, G. M., Harris, M. Y., Zhao, H., & Barbe, M. F. (2016). Manual therapy as an effective treatment for fibrosis in a rat model of upper extremity overuse injury. Journal of the Neurological Sciences, 361, 168-180.

Dilley, A., Richards, N., Pulman, K. G., & Bove, G. M. (2013). Disruption of Fast Axonal Transport in the Rat Induces Behavioral Changes Consistent With Neuropathic Pain. The Journal of Pain, 14(11), 1437-1449.

Fisher, B. E., Southam, A. C., Kuo, Y., Lee, Y., & Powers, C. M. (2016). Evidence of altered corticomotor excitability following targeted activation of gluteus maximus training in healthy individuals. *NeuroReport, 27*(6), 415-421. doi:10.1097

Fisher PW, Zhao Y, Rico MC, Massicotte VS, Wade CK, Litvin J, Bove GM, Popoff SN, Barbe MF. Increased CCN2, substance P and tissue fibrosis are associated with sensorimotor declines in a rat model of repetitive overuse injury. J Cell Commun Signal., 2015 doi: 10.1007/s12079-015-0263-0

Brooks, Vernon B., and W. Thomas Thach. "Cerebellar Control of Posture and Movement." *Comprehensive Physiology* (2011): n. pag. Web.

Brooks, Vernon B. *The Neural Basis of Motor Control*. New York: Oxford UP, 1986. Print.

Brooks, Vernon B: Motor Control How posture and movement are governed. Phys Ther. 1983, 63 (5): 664-673.

Butler, D. S., & Jones, M. A. (1991). *Mobilisation of the nervous system*. Melbourne: Churchill Livingstone.

Butler, D. S., & Moseley, G. L. (2003). *Explain pain*. Adelaide: Noigroup Publications.

Chaitow, L. (2006). *Muscle energy techniques.* Edinburgh: Churchill Livingstone/Elsevier.

Chaitow, L. (2012). The ARTT of palpation? *Journal of Bodywork and Movement Therapies, 16*(2), 129-131. doi:10.1016/j.jbmt.2012.01.018

Cook, G. (2010). *Movement Functional Movement Systems: Screening, Assessment, Corrective Strategies.* Cork: BookBaby.

Davids, K., Bennett, S., & Newell, K. M. (2006). *Movement system variability.* Champaign, IL: Human Kinetics.

Desikachar, T. K. (1999). *The heart of yoga: Developing a personal practice.* Rochester, VT: Inner Traditions International.

Earls, J. *Born to walk: Myofascial efficiency and the body in movement.*

Falsone, Sue. (2014, May 13). East vs. West | Structure & Function. Retrieved November 10, 2014 www.suefalsone.com

Falsone, Sue, "The Thoracic Spine". Retrieved July 02, 2016, from http://movementlectures.com/

Feldenkrais, M. (2002). *The potent self: A study of spontaneity and compulsion.* Berkeley, CA: Frog.

Feldenkrais, M., & Beringer, E. (2010). *Embodied wisdom: The collected papers of Moshe´ Feldenkrais.* San Diego, CA: Somatic Resources.

Flor, H., Braun, C., Elbert, T., & Birbaumer, N. (1997). Extensive reorganization of primary somatosensory cortex in chronic back pain patients. *Neuroscience Letters, 224*(1), 5-8. doi:10.1016/s0304-3940(97)13441-3

Frost, R. (2013). *Applied kinesiology: A training manual and reference book of basic principles and practices.* Berkeley, CA: North Atlantic Books.

Gibbons, J.. *The vital glutes: Connecting the gait cycle to pain and dysfunction.*

Gray, Gary. (2001). *Total body functional profile.* Adrian, MI: Wynn Marketing.

Gray, Gary. *Functional Video Digest Series.* "*Lumbar Spine v. 2.4*" Adrian Michigan, Wynn Marketing

Gray, Gary. *Functional Video Digest Series.* "*Functional Manual Reaction: The Hips v. 3.1*" Adrian Michigan, Wynn Marketing

Gray, Gary. *Functional Video Digest Series.* "*Tweakology v. 3.6*" Adrian Michigan, Wynn Marketing

Grob, K., Ackland, T., Kuster, M., Manestar, M., & Filgueira, L. (2016). A newly discovered muscle: The tensor of the vastus intermedius. *Clin. Anat. Clinical Anatomy, 29*(2), 256-263. doi:10.1002/ca.22680

Hammer, W. I. (1991). *Functional soft tissue examination and treatment by manual methods: The extremities.* Gaithersburg, MD: Aspen.

Hodges, P. W., Butler, J. E., Mckenzie, D. K., & Gandevia, S. C. (1997). Contraction of the human diaphragm during rapid postural adjustments. *The Journal of Physiology, 505*(2), 539-548. doi:10.1111/j.1469-7793.1997.539bb.x

Hodges, P. W., Mellor, R., Crossley, K., & Bennell, K. (2008). Pain induced by injection of hypertonic saline into the infrapatellar fat pad and effect on coordination of the quadriceps muscles. *Arthritis Care & Research Arthritis & Rheumatism, 61*(1), 70-77. doi:10.1002/art.24089

Isaacs, E. R., Bookhout, M. R., & Bourdillon, J. F. (2002). *Bourdillon's spinal manipulation*. Boston: Butterworth-Heinemann.

Iyengar, B. K. (1979). *Light on yoga: Yoga dipika*. New York: Schocken Books.

Järvinen, T. A., Józsa, L., Kannus, P., Järvinen, T. L., & Järvinen, M. (2002, February). Organization and distribution of intramuscular connective tissue in normal and immobilized skeletal muscles. An immunohistochemical, polarization and scanning electron microscopic study. *Journal of Muscle Research and Cell Motility, 23*(3), 245-254. doi:10.1023/a:1020904518336

Kendall, F. P. (1993). *Muscle Testing and Function*. Baltimore, Maryland USA: Williams and Wilkins.

Lewit, Karel, and Sarka Olsanska. "Clinical Importance of Active Scars: Abnormal Scars as a Cause of Myofascial Pain." *Journal of Manipulative and Physiological Therapeutics* 27.6 (2004): 399-402. Web.

Lindsay, Mark, and Chad Robertson. *Fascia: Clinical Applications for Health and Human Performance*. Clifton Park, NY: Delmar, 2008. Print.

Myers, Thomas W. *Anatomy Trains: Myofascial Meridians for Manual and Movement Therapists*. Edinburgh: Churchill Livingstone, 2001. Print.

Nickelston, P., DC. "Take the Brakes off of Movement". Retrieved July 02, 2016, from http://movementlectures.com/

Nijs, Jo, Liesbeth Daenen, Patrick Cras, Filip Struyf, Nathalie Roussel, and Rob A.b. Oostendorp. "Nociception Affects Motor Output." *The Clinical Journal of Pain* 28.2 (2012): 175-81. Web.

Osar, Evan. *Corrective Exercise Solutions to Common Shoulder and Hip Dysfunction*. Cork: BookBaby, 2012. Print.

Page, Phillip, Clare C. Frank, and Robert Lardner. *Assessment and Treatment of Muscle Imbalance: The Janda Approach*. Champaign, IL: Human Kinetics, 2010. Print.

Pearcey, Gregory E. P., David J. Bradbury-Squires, Jon-Erik Kawamoto, Eric J. Drinkwater, David G. Behm, and Duane C. Button. "Foam Rolling for Delayed-Onset Muscle Soreness and Recovery of Dynamic Performance Measures." *Journal of Athletic Training* 50.1 (2015): 5-13. Web.

Pelletier, René, Johanne Higgins, and Daniel Bourbonnais. "Is Neuroplasticity in the Central Nervous System the Missing Link to Our Understanding of Chronic Musculoskeletal Disorders?" *BMC Musculoskeletal Disorders BMC Musculoskelet Disord* 16.1 (2015): 25. Web.

Physiology of the Joints.: Annotated Diagram of the Mechanics of the Human Joints. UK: Churchill Livingstone, 1974. Print.

Rio, Ebonie, Dawson Kidgell, Craig Purdam, Jamie Gaida, G. Lorimer Moseley, Alan J. Pearce, and Jill Cook. "Isometric Exercise Induces Analgesia and Reduces Inhibition in Patellar Tendinopathy." *British Journal of Sports Medicine Br J Sports Med* 49.19 (2015): 1277-283. Web.

Rolf, Ida P. *Rolfing: Reestablishing the Natural Alignment and Structural Integration of the Human Body for Vitality and Well-being.* Rochester, VT: Healing Arts, 1989. Print.

Rolf, Ida P., and Rosemary Feitis. *Rolfing and Physical Reality.* Rochester, VT: Healing Arts, 1990. Print.

Root, M. L., Orien, W. P., & Weed, J. H. (1977). *Normal and abnormal function of the foot.* Los Angeles: Clinical Biomechanics.

Scarr, Graham. *Biotensegrity: The Structural Basis of Life.* Scotland: Handspring, 2014. Print.

Schleip, Robert. "Fascia as an Organ of Communication." *Fascia: The Tensional Network of the Human Body* (2012): 77-79. Web.

Schmidt, Richard A. *Motor Learning and Performance: From Principles to Practice.* Champaign, IL: Human Kinetics ., 1991. Print.

Schultz, R. Louis, and Rosemary Feitis. *The Endless Web: Fascial Anatomy and Physical Reality.* Berkeley, CA: North Atlantic, 1996. Print.

Stecco, Luigi, John V. Basmanjian, and Julie Ann Day. *Fascial Manipulation for Musculoskeletal Pain.* Padova: Piccin, 2004. Print.

Stone, Caroline. *Science in the Art of Osteopathy: Osteopathic Principles and Practice.* Cheltenham: Stanley Thornes, 1999. Print.

Weinstock, David. *NeuroKinetic Therapy: An Innovative Approach to Manual Muscle Testing.* Berkeley, CA: North Atlantic, 2010. Print.

Wolf, C. *Flexibility Highways,* www.HumanMotionAssociates.com

Wolf, C *Flexibility Highways in Motion,* www.HumanMotionAssociates.com

Acknowledgements

Without the support and encouragement of so many people, this work wouldn't have come to fruition.

I've had the opportunity to learn from so many great minds. First, thank you to my patients, who have allowed me to continuously hone my craft, and have provided me with the opportunity to help them feel and move better. Only through their trust and willingness to help me help them have I been able to settle into the clinician and person I am today. Early in life I was taught the importance of regular practice. I remember my Papa Sy saying "practice doesn't make perfect, practice makes better," and while he was talking about golf (he was a golf instructor), it's a mindset I've tried to apply to every practice I sustain. I find joy in practicing my craft regularly, and being able to assist others to enhance their lives. I'm grateful to have discovered personal practices that have allowed me to help myself and help others.

I feel grateful to my parents, Laura and Arnie Kimmel and Chuck and Lauren Wolf, whose approach and different entrepreneurial styles enabled me to develop my talents and thrive in environments that allow me to bring people and ideas together, and this book is proof. I feel lucky to have their support and love.

There have been a number of individuals who have directly influenced my career. Specifically, physical therapist and movement guru Dr. Gary Gray, PT, founder of Applied Functional Science and the Gray Institute. The community in which he built has helped to solidify my approach and understanding of movement, while encouraging me to share my knowledge. It led me to some of my closest friends and guides, including Dr. Nicholas Studholme, DC. His voice, friendship, conversations and demonstrations led me to seek out muscle testing as a tool for my practice, which led me to Neurokinetic Therapy, and the work of David Weinstock, who has become a great resource. The addition of muscle testing and NKT has allowed me to develop into a better clinician, and I'm thankful to these people and so many others for influencing my path.

I also want specifically to thank my father, Chuck Wolf, who is my first mentor and coach. My father has been a continuous resource for me as I've learned movement, and I'm grateful to him for starting me on my path. Thanks Dad.

Other people that deserve mention and have helped me to become the clinician I am today include Dr. David Tiberio, who among other things taught me the importance of asking why, and being very specific in the questions I ask. I'd like to thank Lenny Parracino, who has been a friend and mentor and one of the most gifted bodyworkers and movement minds I know. He taught me the art of reconciling various thought processes and be able to synthesize information to pull out the "truths" in various topics.

I want to thank my uncle Stephen Wolf, who helped me to edit this work and not embarrass myself relative to grammar and English. Thank you David Rich Sol, my friend and publisher who has been so influential in guiding me through this process. He talked me down from the ledge on more than one occasion about quitting on this book, and I wouldn't have been able to complete this project without him. In addition, thank you to Katie Koenig and Amanda Herlihy for taking and editing such great pictures.

Last, I want to thank my beautiful children, Alexia and Elijah. They are my motivation and primary driver in life. They are my greatest teachers, pointing out my flaws and also strengths, and providing me with the ultimate desire to better myself so I can better assist them and others I come into contact with.

Very last, I want to thank my partner and confidant in life, Jessica. She provides me perspective, while inspiring me to be the best person, clinician, father, teacher, mentor and friend I can be. I value her insight and how she encourages me to be better, grounded and confident in myself.

I love you all. And couldn't do this without you and many more. Thank you.

ABOUT THE AUTHOR

Adam's professional credentials include: Licensure in Physical Therapy (IL) and Massage Therapy (IL), Fellow of Applied Functional Science (Gray Institute)(09), Level III practitioner of Neurokinetic Therapy (NKT), Enhance Running Technician, Functional Range Conditioning Practitioner, and has been an Elite Provider of Active Release Technique (ART).

His professional career spans nearly two decades and includes clinical, management, consulting, education, performance/strength and conditioning, as well as ownership roles.

His professional interests lie in a deeper understanding of human movement combined with manual medicine, while creating innovative therapy and business paradigms that facilitate the growth of his patients and colleagues.

Adam regularly presents to fitness and rehabilitation professionals nationally and internationally, and is co-owner of REAL pt, located in Chicago, Illinois.

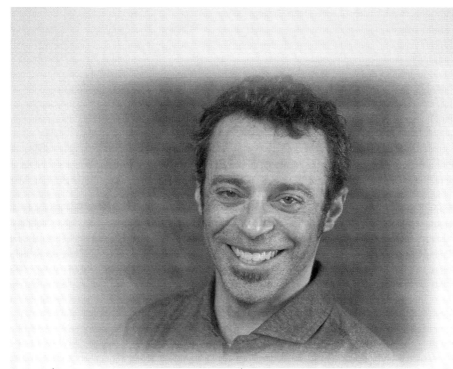

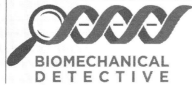

BIOMECHANICAL DETECTIVE

Adam Wolf, PT, LMT, FAFS
Physical Therapist
www.REALmovementPT.com
P/F: 312-489-8579

More information on Adam and his offerings, including educational videos, online courses and live workshops, please visit

www.biomechanicaldetective.com

Be sure to check out the newest video, Improving Fascial Highways: A Perspective on Integrated Motion & Motor Control.

20054761R00106

Printed in Great Britain
by Amazon